Practical Nutrition and Hydration for Dementia-Friendly Mealtimes

of related interest

Essentials of Dementia
Everything You Really Need to Know for Working in Dementia Care
Dr Shibley Rahman and Professor Rob Howard
Forewords by Karen Harrison Dening and Kate Swaffer
ISBN 978 1 78592 397 5
eISBN 978 1 78450 754 1

Sensory Modulation in Dementia Care
Assessment and Activities for Sensory-Enriched Care
Tina Champagne
ISBN 978 1 78592 733 1
eISBN 978 1 78450 427 4

Adaptive Interaction and Dementia
How to Communicate without Speech
Dr Maggie Ellis and Professor Arlene Astell
Illustrated by Suzanne Scott
ISBN 978 1 78592 197 1
eISBN 978 1 78450 471 7

Practical Nutrition and Hydration for Dementia-Friendly Mealtimes

LEE MARTIN

Foreword by Caroline Lecko

Jessica Kingsley *Publishers*
London and Philadelphia

CITY OF KAWARTHA LAKES

First published in 2019
by Jessica Kingsley Publishers
73 Collier Street
London N1 9BE, UK
and
400 Market Street, Suite 400
Philadelphia, PA 19106, USA

www.jkp.com

Library of Congress Cataloging in Publication Data
A CIP catalog record for this book is available from the Library of Congress

British Library Cataloguing in Publication Data
A CIP catalogue record for this book is available from the British Library

ISBN 978 1 84905 700 4
eISBN 978 1 78450 221 8

Printed and bound in the United States

Contents

Foreword

It is with great pleasure that I pen the foreword for this book, having experienced caring for a family member with dementia and so clearly remembering how difficult mealtimes become as our dementia journey progressed.

Despite my many years of experience as a nurse I did not feel equipped to support my relative with dementia or my family to provide the nutritional care that was needed as we faced behavioural changes, food preference changes and latterly swallowing difficulties – challenges that I now know so many families and carers struggle with. The challenges that we faced were not just around our own lack of knowledge and experience in caring for a person with dementia, but also with the amazing care staff who really struggled to cope at mealtimes with people with dementia.

The chapters within this book provide much-needed practical solutions to improve the mealtime experience, nutrition and hydration for people living with dementia. Key to this is using the Dementia Mealtime Assessment Tool as a resource for assessing and monitoring mealtimes, and the evidence-based interventions will provide you with a range of tools to help you in providing person-centred care to support mealtimes for people with advancing dementia.

I believe that we all take the ability to eat and drink for granted – as a necessary thing to do – that is, until we or someone we love is unable to do so. It is, perhaps, then and only then that we appreciate that eating and drinking is not simply something we do; it is so much more.

I am delighted that this book has been published as I believe that it will provide a valuable resource for carers who are required to provide this highly complex care at mealtimes for people with dementia.

Caroline Lecko
Nutrition and Hydration Week co-lead

1

Dementia and Mealtimes

Introduction

For many people living with dementia, as the disease progresses to the later stages, they become increasingly dependent on carers. Often people with later-stage dementia require additional care in their own home or when this becomes too complex require increased care in care homes.

Providing support with eating and drinking can be the most time-intensive caring role, as clearly most people need to eat a few times each day with meals taking time to be consumed (Aselage, Amella and Watson, 2011). The actual mealtime involves a complex mix of environmental, social, cultural, physical and supportive caring factors, which all impact on the ability of a person with dementia to be able to consume enough to meet their basic nutritional requirements. Aside from nutrition, mealtimes also provide an opportunity for socialising and engaging with others.

As dementia progresses a reduction in eating abilities and behaviours at mealtimes is observed and the complexities of nutritional care become more difficult for the carer. Faced with this complex situation carers tend to rely on past clinical experiences mixed with personal beliefs to determine appropriate interventions. Without appropriate knowledge and skills, however, this can lead to carers misinterpreting someone's eating and drinking abilities and behaviours at mealtimes, and not really knowing how to effectively support them (Batchelor-Murphy et al., 2015a). For example, someone staring at their food without eating, or becoming agitated at a mealtime, may be misinterpreted as a sign of not wanting to eat rather than as a sign that a loss of abilities needed at mealtimes (in combination with an unsupportive mealtime environment) is preventing them from eating independently. This loss of independence often means the carer takes over the mealtime role and feeds the person, which fosters dependence and may not improve nutritional intake. The consequences of this are published widely in the research literature with many people with dementia experiencing weight loss, dehydration, malnutrition, unnecessary enteral tube feeding, loss of independence and dignity and decreased quality of life. The many common reduced mealtime abilities and behaviours which are described in this book are often not recognised or understood by the carer or indeed the family members. The family visiting their parent in a care home for example may in fact accuse the carers of not taking nutritional care of their loved one.

Carers may not even be aware of the many practical and evidence-based interventions that can be put in place to support the person to maintain mealtime independence for longer. Appropriate observation and assessment of an individual's mealtime abilities can help design a person-centred care plan to support the retained eating abilities and enhance nutritional intake independently. There is a range of practical evidence-based interventions that can be applied to the mealtime setting to improve nutritional intake but unfortunately current nutrition and dementia guidelines hardly mention them (Volkert et al., 2015). Despite this, much research is continuing to highlight the importance of supporting people with advancing dementia more appropriately at mealtimes and hopefully guidelines will eventually follow. Until such time it is important for carers to be aware of the many practical intervention options they have to add to their mealtime caring skills.

There is a pressing need to improve mealtime care for people with dementia, particularly for those living in the moderate to later stages. Requests from carers for advice and support with nutrition and hydration concerns are particularly related to the management of eating abilities and meal behaviours (Prince et al., 2014). This book provides an informal educational tool regarding eating abilities and meal behaviours as dementia advances, the aim being to help support mealtime independence for as long as possible.

Dementia
Context
Dementia is an umbrella term that describes a set of symptoms including memory loss, confusion, problems communicating and reasoning, and

mood and behaviour changes (Department of Health, 2015). Dementia is caused by damage to the brain by many different diseases and in some cases a combination of more than one. The most common types are Alzheimer's disease, vascular dementia, frontotemporal dementia and dementia with Lewy bodies. Dementia is a progressive disease, meaning symptoms get worse over time. Whatever form of dementia someone has it affects people differently and the level of support required will vary. Most important is to recognise that no two people with dementia are the same, and individuals will have unique and differing needs (DHSC and AHPPU, 2016).

Dementia is a major contributor to disability, dependence and transition from living at home to living in care facilities such as care homes. In the later stages behavioural and psychological symptoms of dementia (BPSD) increase and impact on the quality of life of both the person with dementia and their carer(s) (Prince *et al.*, 2014).

Prevalence

- The number of people living with dementia worldwide is currently estimated at 47 million (as of 2015) and is projected to increase to 75 million by 2030. The number of cases of dementia are estimated to almost triple by 2050 to 132 million. A new diagnosis of dementia is made every three seconds based on 9.9 million new cases of dementia per year. In 2015 the total global societal cost of dementia was estimated to be US$818 billion, up from US$604 billion in 2010. This corresponds to 1.1 per cent of the worldwide gross domestic product (GDP) (WHO, 2017).

- In the UK 850,000 people live with dementia (as of 2015); this includes over 700,000 people in England. Over 40,000 younger people in the UK (65 years of age or below) have dementia, and an estimated 25,000 people from Black, Asian and minority ethnic groups have the condition. The overall number is set to rise to one million by 2021 and over two million by 2051 (Kane and Terry, 2015).

- The ever-increasing numbers of dementia population statistics such as those provided by the Alzheimer's Society above are, however, disputed in the research. According to research by the Medical Research Council (MRC) the UK has seen a 20 per cent fall in the incidence of dementia over the past two decades. For the UK the authors estimate 209,600 new dementia cases per year compared to an anticipated 250,000 new cases based on previous levels (Matthews *et al.*, 2016).

- The number of people living with dementia is set to increase as our population ages. The prevalence of dementia increases with age in that 6 to 14 per cent of over-65-year-olds have dementia, while this increases to over 30 per cent for those over 85 years old and over 37 per cent in those 90 and over. Therefore the older you get the higher the risk of getting dementia (Sura *et al.*, 2012). Dementia though is not necessarily an inevitable part of ageing. Although dementia mainly affects older people it can start before the age of 65 and in this case is termed young onset dementia.

Impact

- Dementia and Alzheimer's disease have replaced ischaemic heart diseases as the leading cause of death in England and Wales, accounting for 11.6 per cent of all deaths registered in 2015 (ONS, 2017). The Office for National Statistics says the change is largely due to an ageing population: people are living for longer and deaths from some other causes, including heart disease, have gone down. Also, doctors have got better at diagnosing dementia and the condition is now given more importance on death certificates.

- The annual cost of dementia to society in the UK is estimated at £26.3 billion. This corresponds to an average cost per person of £32,250 annually including £5300 in health care and £12,500 in social care costs (Public Health England, 2016). The vast majority of these costs are borne by the families of people living with dementia and this seems to be the same worldwide. Specifically looking at costs associated with 560 people with dementia a Spanish study concluded that the monthly overall mean cost of Alzheimer's disease was

1412.73 euros. Almost 88 per cent of these costs was funded by the patient's own family, adding a financial burden to these families (Coduras *et al.*, 2010).

- There are currently around 670,000 carers of people with dementia in the UK. Caring for a person with dementia is unlike caring for a person with any other condition, and many carers will experience high levels of stress and even depression (Kane and Terry, 2015). It is estimated that 66,000 carers have cut their working hours to make time for caring, while 50,000 people have left work altogether (DHSC and AHPPU, 2016).

- In the UK one in four hospital beds are occupied by people with dementia. This accounted for 3.2 million bed days in 2013/14 (Kane and Terry, 2015).

- Care homes remain the largest institutional settings in the UK where people with dementia receive care, including a third of all people with dementia. Generally in care homes up to 70 per cent of care home residents in the UK have dementia or significant memory problems. Care homes are also the setting where the majority of people with dementia reach the end of their lives (Kane and Terry, 2015).

- An important report on nutrition and dementia highlights the lack of importance and attention directed towards nutrition and malnutrition seen in people living with dementia (Prince *et al.*, 2014). Evidence suggests that 20 to 45 per cent of people living with dementia in the community have significant weight loss and 50 per cent in care homes have inadequate food intake. Reasons for weight loss and reduced food intake are complex, with many of these complex problems manifesting as changes in mealtime eating abilities and meal behaviours.

- Weight loss in dementia is associated with greater dependence needs through reduced functional abilities and worsening symptoms of dementia. Weight loss in combination with these factors increases the risk of morbidity, hospitalisation, institutionalisation and early mortality (Prince *et al.*, 2014).

Signs, symptoms and stages

Dementia affects each person in a different way, depending upon the impact and type of the disease and the person's personality before becoming ill. The signs and symptoms linked to dementia can be understood in three stages linked to the severity of the disease. Clinically the stages of dementia are determined using assessment tools measuring cognitive impairment, for example: the Mini-Mental State Examination (MMSE), Global Deterioration scale (GDS) or Clinical Dementia Rating (CDR) (Abdelhamid *et al.*, 2016). These assessment tools provide a score which will then determine what level of cognitive impairment and what severity of dementia the person has. There are typically four different categories as shown in Table 1.1 but around the world different words are used to describe the stages of dementia.

Table 1.1: The clinical stages of dementia

Clinical stage[1]	Alzheimer's Australia (Alzheimer's Australia, 2017)	Alzheimer's Association (America)[2] (Alzheimer's Association, 2017)
Mild cognitive impairment	Not applicable	Not applicable
Mild dementia	Early	Mild (early stage)
Moderate dementia	Moderate	Moderate (middle stage)
Severe dementia	Advanced	Severe (late stage)

1   Clinical stage based on assessment tools (MMSE, CDR, GDS).
2   The Alzheimer's Association uses these terms to describe the stages of Alzheimer's rather than the broader term of dementia.

The early or mild stage of dementia is often overlooked, because the onset is gradual. As dementia progresses to moderate or middle stage, the signs and symptoms become clearer and more restricting. Finally in severe/advanced (or late-stage) dementia, memory disturbances are serious and the physical signs and symptoms become more obvious.

You may also come across the stages of dementia described simply as early or later stages, particularly in the UK as seen on the NHS Choices (NHS Choices, 2015) or the Alzheimer's Society websites (Alzheimer's Society, 2017). This is likely a more practical way of describing how dementia progresses and the term 'later-stage' dementia will be referred to throughout the book.

Categorising people with dementia into what symptoms and stage they are at is a very medical and research-based way of understanding things. Certainly as dementia advances people may display mid- and late-stage functions within the same day or even within the same hour. Therefore it is better to assess the person as they present themselves each day rather than relying on the stages of dementia.

One of the main issues with categories is that they may ignore the abilities that are still present and foster dependence rather than supporting and preserving abilities. This is excellently described by dementia campaigner Beth Britton on her blog, where she writes, among other words of wisdom, that a person with dementia needs appropriate care and support and not a misleading label (Britton, 2015).

There are a couple of excellent 'mantras' that relate to this and summarise the above in a few words: 'Look at the person not the dementia!' and 'See the ME in deMEntia.'

Often in clinical practice the carer or health professional does not have detail of the type of dementia let alone the symptoms or severity stage at which the person is defined as being (Tristani, 2016). Research always tries to define the severity so the success of interventions can be applied to the correct stage. As mentioned however, as the symptoms of dementia can change daily it is unwise to only adopt certain interventions for certain stages of dementia. If we take Alzheimer's disease as an example, we know that for approximately 40 per cent of the time (four years), someone with Alzheimer's experiences the most severe stage of the disease (Arrighi *et al.*, 2010). As dementia progresses to a more advanced stage this often leads to increased care needs and the person entering a care home. Therefore for the vast majority of people in a care home with dementia it is the more severe stage and more severe symptoms carers will encounter. In terms of mealtimes and dementia we can assume that when someone is no longer able to self-feed then this is a sign they have entered into the later stages of the disease (Tristani, 2016).

In this book the vast majority of information is based on research evidence and as such will categorise people into the three stages discussed. The book is designed to support people with what would be classed as the later stages (moderate to severe) of dementia.

Dementia language

Language guidelines are focused on empowering people with dementia and removing stigma, as the quote above highlights. The language used in this book has attempted to follow the guidelines set out in the publication 'Dementia Words Matter: Guidelines on language about dementia', a collaboration by the Dementia Action Alliance, and the Dementia Engagement and Empowerment Project (DEEP) (DEEP, 2014). The guidelines also use Alzheimer's Australia 'Dementia Language Guidelines' (2015). These guidelines encourage the focus of language on the abilities rather than the deficits of people living with dementia. You may therefore read words used in this book that you do not read in the research on the topic involved. Where applicable this will be highlighted and Chapter 2 in particular highlights issues with the language previously used in research to describe 'difficulties' experienced by people with dementia at mealtimes. The aim of the language in the book is to help you understand that creating a supportive mealtime is one of the key points in improving nutrition and hydration. Using words such as 'supportive' and 'abilities' rather than 'problems' or 'difficulties' should help you see a different way of looking at the person with dementia.

Inappropriate use of language can stigmatise the person with dementia, and the nutritional care of people with dementia could also be associated with stigma. For example you may assume that weight loss and not eating or drinking is a normal part of dementia progressing. This stigma may reduce the type, amount or quality of care provided to a person with advancing dementia and therefore no positive changes will be made (Swaffer, 2014).

Person-centred care

Person-centred care involves tailoring a person's care to their interests, abilities, history and personality (Alzheimer's Society, 2009). This is one of many definitions of person-centred care and put simply it places the person at the centre of care. Another definition is that person-centred care is a best-practice approach that supports individuals holistically and respects personal abilities, values, preferences and needs (Hung, Chaudhury and Rust, 2016), aiming to improve quality of life (Chaudhury, Hung and Badger, 2013).

This book aims to promote a practical application of person-centred care, in that the practical assessment of the person with dementia at a mealtime takes into account their needs, preferences and strengths while the practical interventions are harmonised and tailored to those particular needs, preferences and strengths.

Throughout the book I will try to convey the evidence behind person-centred assessment and interventions in a way that ensures people with dementia are always treated with dignity, compassion and respect. Focusing on their strengths and abilities (mealtime abilities) – not deficits (feeding difficulties) – at mealtimes will ensure that a person-centred approach is adopted at each mealtime and independence rather than dependence is promoted.

Recently a person-centred care model focusing on nutrition care for people with dementia in care homes has been proposed with a focus on supporting mealtime abilities (Murphy, Holmes and Brooks, 2017). This paper provides a much-needed outline of the main themes that are required for a person-centred care process including providing appropriate support, choice, environment, socialisation, carer interaction and resources to guide nutritional care. In this book it is hoped the practical application of these important person-centred themes can be provided to allow carers to implement a person-centred nutritional care approach at every mealtime. This will often require a shift in attitudes, culture and organisational practices moving away from the traditional 'task-focused' model of care to a person-centred care model (Chaudhury et al., 2013).

Dementia and mealtimes

To help set the scene surrounding the interventions required to better support people with dementia at mealtimes a brief overview of some key research evidence is provided.

Research overview

Since the mid-2000s there have been a number of literature reviews discussing the evidence for interventions that improve nutrition-related outcomes (e.g. increased food intake, weight, BMI). For people living with moderate to severe dementia the literature evidence focuses on eating abilities and meal behaviours, referred to collaboratively in this book as mealtime abilities. One of the first review papers highlighted three themes which have continued to be highlighted in subsequent research (Watson and Green, 2006).

1. It is unlikely that one single intervention will be effective in improving nutrition outcomes.

2. There is a lack of assessment completed for measuring mealtime abilities.

3. There is a need to link effective interventions to specific mealtime abilities.

Further reviews of the research evidence supported the conclusions of these original authors, once again highlighting that multicomponent interventions targeted at supporting mealtime abilities would be the best approach for improving nutrition-related health outcomes (Liu, Cheon and Thomas, 2014). There is evidence that multicomponent interventions using improved socialisation at mealtimes, appropriate tableware and environmental adjustments can be associated with increased energy intake and body weight (Prince *et al.*, 2014). The importance of multicomponent interventions in having a greater benefit on improved nutritional outcomes has also been highlighted in scoping reviews of the research literature, which can provide a look at a broader range of topics compared to a specific research question used when completing a systematic review (Vucea, Keller and Ducak, 2014).

A group of researchers produced two systematic reviews in 2013 and 2014. The first looked more broadly at the entire mealtime experience, that is, from changing food service provision to environmental adaptations at mealtimes. They found that simple interventions based on these aspects can improve outcomes such as increased food intake (Abbott *et al.*, 2013). Their following study focused specifically on BPSD, or as this book describes them, 'meal behaviours'. The systematic review found that simple, cost-effective interventions aimed at creating a supportive mealtime environment can improve meal behaviour symptoms (Whear *et al.*, 2014).

Finally other narrative reviews have focused on the neglected topic of the psychosocial aspects of mealtimes which can improve both food intake and quality of life. The author highlights the importance of this along with the need for a range of interventions that address the many diverse components associated with mealtimes for persons with dementia (Keller, 2016).

Interest in the topics of mealtime experience, mealtime environment, psychosocial aspects of mealtimes and multicomponent interventions targeted at supporting mealtime abilities continues to grow with another extensive systematic literature review due to be completed by the Cochrane reviews (Herke *et al.*, 2015).

The current theme emerging from research is the use of a multicomponent intervention approach to nutritional dementia care. As anyone working in dementia care will know, there is not one solution for one person: a range of different interventions for different individuals is required.

Research limitations

The book is not designed to provide another in-depth review of the research evidence as highlighted above. This is much better performed by academics in research institutions. The book will, however, focus on the practical application of the evidence and not dwell on the limitations of research designs. All the evidence discussed in the reviews mentioned above and throughout the book have several limitations, and the reader should be referred to the full research papers for a detailed critical appraisal. In general the nutrition-related outcomes such as increases in food intake, weight or calorific content are limited by the quality of the study design and methodology used (Watson and Green, 2006; Abbott *et al.*, 2013; Liu *et al.*, 2014; Whear *et al.*, 2014; Volkert *et al.*, 2015). A lack of randomised controlled trials also limits the strength of evidence for interventions – especially when conducting systematic reviews.

This is why you may read systematic reviews of evidence on all aspects of mealtime dementia care that point to 'no evidence' or a 'lack of effectiveness' for successful interventions (Abdelhamid *et al.*, 2016). When assessed against robust research methodologies and designs the studies do not meet high-quality standards. This may be a case of 'absence of evidence' rather than 'evidence of absence' of effective interventions (Prince *et al.*, 2014).

Regardless, carers are required to provide 'high-quality' care in the midst of this apparent lack of effective solutions. Indeed low-quality evidence does not mean interventions will not be effective for some individuals. As everyone with dementia is an individual then what works for one person may not work for another (Stone, 2014). You can read the research to work out possible interventions but in reality what works in research may not work in a real-life setting. In research you have to control variables affecting what you are measuring, which may mean complex interactions are not fully understood. In real life you cannot prevent giving an intervention to someone because they display other variables that may affect the effectiveness of your intervention. Perhaps this is partly why this area of care is so poorly understood and why there is a lack of information on what interventions carers can specifically implement to support people living with dementia at mealtimes.

This book delves into the practicalities of the current research to identify interventions that can work and that focus on improving independence, quality of life and nutritional intake. One aim of the book is to provide carers with a set of practical interventions to help with the complexities of mealtimes.

Practical application

Looking at the evidence provided by research gives us a starting point but translating that evidence into practical and usable daily caring strategies requires more thought. The aim of this book is to translate the research evidence into a practical model of care centred on the mealtime. Mealtime care is complex and to help translate all the complexities in practice means using a structured and systematic approach. This of course must still be flexible to bend with the needs of the person. This is why a person-centred approach with a focus on independence, dignity and quality of life (rather than an over-reliance on more traditional outcomes such as weight and body mass index (BMI) measurements) will help achieve a better mealtime experience for the person with dementia and their carer.

The vast majority of research has been conducted on people with dementia in long-term care; however, many of the findings are generalisable to home care by informal and unpaid carers (Prince *et al.*, 2014).

Purpose of the book

In general the nutritional care for people with dementia has focused first on nutrition support techniques such as food fortification, eating little and often and providing medical nutrition such as oral nutrition supplements. These interventions are designed to enhance the macro- and micronutrient content of foods eaten; however, they provide little encouragement for people with dementia to actually eat. Typically this advice follows a standard assessment of the person with dementia using measurement of weight, BMI and so on, or screening questionnaires (e.g. the Malnutrition Universal Screening Tool, MUST). Nutrition support interventions based on these typical assessments are clearly important but they only form a part of the solution to improved nutrition and hydration care for people with dementia. Nutrition support interventions do not help overcome the common barriers to sufficient nutritional intake such as reduced mealtime abilities.

Perhaps more important than these traditional nutrition support interventions is the use of a range of multicomponent interventions all designed to better support the independence of the person with dementia at mealtimes. It certainly makes sense in a disease such as dementia, where changes in the abilities required to eat and drink along with behaviours at mealtimes both prevent nutritional intake; interventions aimed at supporting these abilities will be the most beneficial.

To create a range of multicomponent interventions however, we must first start using different types of assessment tools, which are discussed in Chapter 3. A carer needs to be able to identify the current strengths a person has at the mealtime in regard to their eating, drinking and meal behaviours and abilities. The carer can then further support these strengths and enhance reduced mealtime abilities using a set of multicomponent interventions including cueing techniques, modifying the table setting and tableware, improving familiarity, increasing socialisation and adapting the mealtime environment. All of these interventions are designed to simplify and enhance the mealtime experience, allowing the person with dementia to eat independently for as long as possible. Certainly recent research is reaffirming what this book details: that there are many areas of mealtime care that need to be combined to provide person-centred care (Murphy et al., 2017).

Supporting the eating and drinking abilities and meal behaviours of people with dementia can be daunting for both paid and unpaid carers (Aselage et al., 2011). As dementia progresses individuals may forget to eat or forget they have eaten, seemingly fail to recognise food or the mealtime setting, have reduced abilities needed to physically eat and drink, and experience increased stress and anxiety at mealtimes. It is important carers are able to assess and intervene appropriately (Aselage, Amella and Watson, 2011) and provide person-centred care.

The way mealtime care is provided for many people with mid- to later-stage dementia requires a reversal of the current traditional process of interventions, where first we must support the person with dementia to continue to eat and drink independently and then adapt the food for nutrition support advice. There is no point adding more and more calories to a food if it is still not eaten. Finally after implementing these interventions first and as dementia becomes more severe then increased carer assistance and feeding are considered.

Therefore rather than focusing on what specific nutrients to provide, this book will deal with the practical application of supporting people with dementia at mealtimes. The correct level of support can not only improve the mealtime experience but also improve health outcomes such as increased food intake, weight gain and quality of life.

The care at mealtimes is complex and often carers receive little or no training on how to specifically manage and support people with dementia at mealtimes. The training that is usually provided focuses frequently on correct positioning and feeding practices, which are important but only part of mealtime care and not applicable to everyone's needs. This results in carers having to learn 'on the job' from their colleagues or on their own (Aselage et al., 2011). It is likely many carers will not know about the extensive range of person-centred interventions that could be adapted for the person they care for. Carers lack access to specific tools and interventions to help them support people with dementia at mealtimes. Training and education for health and social care professionals, paid and unpaid carers and catering teams are essential to meet the complex challenges people with dementia face. Unfortunately the majority of people with dementia are either cared for at home by unpaid carers or in care homes where there is a lack of training, access and funding for the carers in these settings. There is a clear need to educate carers in supporting mealtime abilities (Prince et al., 2014) but this is also applicable to dietitians and other health professionals.

Focus of the book

One aim of the book is to provide carers with a set of practical interventions to help with the complexities of mealtimes.

The focus of the book is to take carers through an evidence-based and structured way to assess the mealtime abilities a person with dementia has retained (or seen a reduction of) and choose appropriate interventions to support and preserve these abilities or enhance reduced abilities. The aim of this is to help the person with dementia to maintain independence and dignity at mealtimes for as long as possible so they can continue to eat and drink, maintain adequate nutrition and have a better quality of life. Quality of life in particular declines as dementia advances and risks of malnutrition increase. Previous independence is replaced by dependence for many daily activities, including eating and drinking. The longer that mealtime abilities can be preserved the better a person's quality of life can be. The book will also emphasise the non-nutrition importance of mealtimes for people with dementia, including social, cultural and psychological factors.

This book will aim to provide more specific guidance at mealtimes and the resources available to help achieve this. A structured observational measure called the Dementia Mealtime Assessment Tool (DMAT) will be used as a practical way to assess mealtime abilities. In each practical chapter an extensive range of evidence-based interventions to choose from will be provided in order to support the identified mealtime ability.

Before this there will be an explanation of mealtime abilities in relation to dementia along with the ways of assessing of mealtime abilities. Separating each practical intervention chapter will be a chapter looking at the evidence behind the suggested interventions, with a focus on the practical aspects of this research evidence.

The book will focus on research evidence conducted in care homes as this is where the majority of dementia mealtime research has taken place. The vast majority of interventions studied in care homes can be replicated in home care. Hospital and acute care will not be covered specifically in this book; however, again, many of the interventions discussed can be applied to the acute setting.

This book does not have the capacity to discuss end-of-life care in dementia or the specific use of medical nutrition including enteral tube feeding. It is however worth remembering that approximately half of people living in a care home die within a year of admission. The mealtime experience and the social interaction provided can therefore play a major role in the quality of life provided in this last year of life (Stone, 2014).

2

Mealtime Abilities in Dementia

Introduction

Mealtimes not only offer nutrition and hydration essential for life but also provide a chance to socialise and offer the opportunity for a sensory experience. As dementia advances however, the ability to feed oneself and socially interact at mealtimes can become a highly complex task (Slaughter *et al.*, 2011). The ability to eat is identified as an activity of daily living (or ADL) and commonly can be one of the last ADLs to be lost in people with dementia as the disease advances (Chang and Roberts, 2008; Aselage and Amella, 2010; Aselage *et al.*, 2011). This lost ability to eat can first cause decreased food intake, followed by loss of body weight (Lin, Watson and Wu, 2010), leading to malnutrition and associated reduced quality of life (Vogelzang, 2003) and contributing to early mortality (Chang and Roberts, 2008; Aselage and Amella, 2010). Therefore the ability to eat is central to self-care and independence, and having this autonomy can help enhance quality of life (Lee and Song, 2015). Some theorise that the ADL of eating is ingrained in the long-term memory and because of this should be seen as a strength that can be retained. It is important to note that lost mealtime abilities can be reacquired when the right environment and cueing are provided (Coyne and Hoskins, 1997).

Interestingly even older people without dementia who restrict their food options due to eating difficulties and physical dependency have an increased risk of malnutrition (Maitre *et al.*, 2014). Clearly if eating difficulties have an impact on older people without dementia then for those with dementia these issues can further expose their vulnerability to weight loss and malnutrition.

Defining mealtime eating abilities and behaviours

There have been many different terms for defining eating abilities and behaviours at mealtimes. Originally the term 'aversive feeding behaviours' was commonly used (Watson, 1996) and mainly described the difficulties encountered by nurses when feeding people with dementia. Both 'feeding difficulty' and 'eating difficulty' were used interchangeably in the research literature (Chang and Roberts, 2008) and usually referred to either the difficulty in feeding a person with dementia or the difficulties they had feeding themselves. Some authors argued that 'feeding difficulties' are different to 'eating difficulties' as feeding involves a direct interface between the carer and the person with dementia, while feeding difficulties should reflect this interaction (Chang and Roberts, 2008). They state that a feeding difficulty provides more information to the carer about what feeding intervention they should be implementing rather than an eating difficulty the person with dementia presents with. Either way, when defining an 'eating or feeding difficulty' this usually involved some key components (Chang and Roberts, 2008):

1.   ability to recognise food and eating utensils

2.   ability to use these utensils to move food from plate to mouth

3.   ability to effectively control chewing and swallowing of food.

There were other terms used and included substituting the word 'difficulty' with 'behaviour', for example 'eating or feeding behaviour'. These terms will be mentioned in this chapter when describing prevalence studies and in the following chapter when discussing assessment tools that measure these concepts at mealtimes. The word 'behaviour' was often used to describe both issues with eating or self-feeding as defined in the three stages above but also to describe other behaviours not related to the physical effort of feeding oneself.

Having all these different terms often meaning the same or very similar thing is clearly confusing. One author who wrote a great deal on this subject set out to clarify them and suggested the term 'mealtime difficulties' be used to refer to the domains of eating, feeding and behaviours observed in older adults with dementia (Aselage, 2010). The author in fact went further and suggested the term should also be considered within the mealtime environment and social implications at mealtimes. Therefore within the overarching term of 'mealtime difficulties', 'feeding behaviours' were used to describe observations seen when a person with dementia was being assisted to eat by a carer, while 'eating behaviours' described both physical and social activity encompassing a variety of 'behaviours' that affected nutritional intake and independence. Finally 'meal behaviours' included elements from 'eating and feeding behaviours' and also included the environmental and social aspects of a mealtime.

The main issue with these previous definitions and terms is that the majority focused on the problem of eating, or indeed being fed, rather than the abilities that could be supported and maintained. This was born out of the need to identify these difficulties and to create assessment tools to measure them (Aselage *et al.*, 2011) which are discussed in the next chapter.

Recent research, and certainly the focus of this book, is on interventions to alleviate the complexities of mealtimes. The mealtime itself is being viewed from a more theoretical viewpoint as the influence of the environment and psychosocial, cultural and personal factors are considered (Aselage *et al.*, 2011). Currently, and rightly so, there is a renewed push to adopt a strength-focused health and social care culture. This means instead of seeing the person with dementia as needing dependence – having many things wrong with them which need to be fixed – we see them as someone with reduced and retainable abilities that can be supported to enhance their independence, using a person-centred approach. Interestingly in one study, once carers were trained to realise 'feeding behaviours' should not be viewed as 'aversive' or 'resistive' but rather as a form of communication – an unmet need – then the carers reacted more positively to these observations by spending more time providing support, which led to increased food intake (Batchelor-Murphy *et al.*, 2015a).

Both 'eating difficulties' and 'feeding difficulties', along with most of the other previously used terms, are no longer preferred although you will still see them being used, especially in research, owing to the history of their use as described above. The following terms of 'eating abilities' and 'meal behaviours' are suggested for clarification and to help the adoption of this caring approach focusing on person-centred care.

Eating abilities

Eating abilities should be considered the preferred term to describe the previous terms of 'feeding and eating difficulties'. Generally defining eating abilities is still based around the three key components of eating mentioned above: recognising food, getting food from the plate to the mouth and swallowing. Therefore in general an eating ability involves the physical movements of eating and would for example mean that if a person with dementia uses the wrong end of a spoon to try to eat they have a reduced eating ability. Explaining to this person that they are using the wrong end of the cutlery or providing them with adapted cutlery (with a spoon head at one end and a fork on the other end) may enhance this eating ability and they can continue to eat independently. This type of eating ability clearly affects the 'ability to feed oneself' and involves the process of bringing food from the plate to the mouth, which is the second concept of the process of eating described above. Other eating abilities are focused on the next stage of eating where you chew and swallow the food. If a swallowing difficulty is identified then the person with dementia will also have a reduced eating ability or more precisely a reduced 'oral ability' to eat.

As there are many different types of eating abilities which affect different parts of the three key concepts in eating, the eating abilities have been separated into categories by all researchers on this subject. In the two examples just given there is the 'ability to self-feed' and 'oral abilities'. Categorising eating abilities like this makes it easier to assess abilities and plan interventions.

Eating abilities do affect the ability to eat and drink but there are also many behaviours that do the same but are more difficult to define using the three key concepts of eating. Consideration needs to be given to environmental, social and cultural factors (Aselage and Amella, 2010) that affect mealtime behaviours which then impact upon eating abilities. For example, someone with dementia may be perfectly able to pick up their cutlery and start eating but the amount of noise and stimulus in the mealtime environment leaves them distracted from the task at hand. They may struggle to start eating and are observed by carers as displaying meal behaviours such as 'Staring at their food' or seeming 'distracted'. Does this then mean they do not recognise the food or cutlery? You cannot be sure unless you intervene. If you provide a more supportive environment by reducing factors that affect their meal behaviours, by reducing noise and distractions, and that person starts to eat independently, then you have enhanced their eating ability and reduced their behavioural symptoms.

Meal behaviours

The example given above describes a distractible behaviour; however, many behaviours observed at mealtimes in people with dementia fall into the domains of agitation, restlessness, being impatient or resisting care. Mealtime behavioural symptoms can prevent someone eating, interrupt others at the meal setting and be distressing to others. One study found the most common observed behaviours at mealtimes in nursing home residents were verbal refusal of care, verbal disruptions and physical refusal of care, for example pushing away (Gilmore-Bykovskyi, 2015). There are several theoretical frameworks to explain behaviours in people living with dementia, for example the Need-Driven Dementia-Compromised Behaviour Model (Algase et al., 1996). The theory most often quoted in literature related to mealtime behaviours is the 'unmet needs' model (Cohen-Mansfield, 2000). Quite simply this suggests that a behaviour is a direct result of a need going unmet; for example the person feels in discomfort so expresses agitation. Certainly when carers have been interviewed they have thought that eating behaviours are an expression of needs (Hsiao, Chao and Wang, 2013).

Other models theorise that behaviours are a response to stimuli in the environment, which include their carers, and that people with dementia have a lower threshold to these stimuli, which then manifest as behaviours. Someone's mealtime needs can go unmet if their senses and level of cognition are over- or under-stimulated and this involves a mix of environmental, social, cultural and personal factors. As the mealtime care of people with dementia is so complex, elements from all the theoretical frameworks are probably relevant to individuals but no one model is specific to everyone. The 'unmet needs' model is perhaps the most relevant to health care as it presents a more person-centred approach, effectively saying that a behaviour indicates the person is not being supported fully and this is not their fault, signifying an intervention can be put in place to improve the situation. Further work based around this unmet-needs model highlights that people in the later stages of dementia can express their needs behaviourally in a non-normative manner rather than verbally. This makes it difficult for carers to understand what their needs are. If these needs are not met it can result in further need and more behaviours expressed, making the carer's job even more complex (Kovach *et al.*, 2005).

Eating abilities and meal behaviours, although different from each other, are intertwined, both affecting the ability to consume food and fluid. For example if a person living with advanced dementia spits out their food it may be because they cannot chew or swallow the food. This is an example of a reduced eating ability or more specifically a reduced 'oral eating ability'. It may however also indicate that the person with dementia does not like the food because of 'personal preference'. Owing to their advanced dementia they cannot verbalise their displeasure and this then becomes an example of a 'meal behaviour'. Behaviours are also often referred to as BPSDs (behavioural and psychological symptoms of dementia); however, for the purpose of this book the term 'meal behaviours' is preferred.

To conclude therefore, when we observe a behaviour at a meal that is affecting a person's nutritional intake and social interaction, interventions that can create a supportive mealtime environment and take account of personal preferences may reduce the behaviour and meet the person's needs. This is further discussed in Chapters 10 and 6 respectively.

Mealtime abilities

The term 'mealtime difficulties' was used to encompass all complexities at a mealtime (Aselage and Amella, 2010). Considering the evaluation of this term and current use of language (DEEP, 2014; Alzheimer's Australia, 2015) this book will use the term 'mealtime abilities' to describe both 'meal behaviours' and 'eating abilities' pertinent to mealtimes. Later in the book when discussing interventions for enhancing abilities and creating a supportive mealtime environment, specific eating abilities and behaviours will be identified so specific interventions can be implemented.

Behaviours may present as a separate set of symptoms from eating abilities but behaviours do affect eating abilities and lead to the same negative health consequences. Therefore when considering nutritional care we need to look at the abilities at mealtimes as a whole and not isolate one from the other (Aselage and Amella, 2010). Drawing on previous work (Chang and Roberts, 2008), recent research

(Liu *et al.*, 2014; Abdelhamid *et al.*, 2016; Murphy *et al.*, 2017) and current dementia language and guidelines (DEEP, 2014; Swaffer, 2014; Alzheimer's Australia, 2015), a new conceptual model for describing the complexities at mealtimes is provided in Figure 2.1.

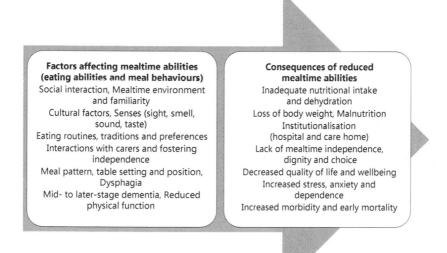

Figure 2.1: *Conceptual model of factors affecting mealtime abilities and consequences of a reduction in these abilities*

In this conceptual model, mealtime abilities are affected by many factors including those present at the mealtime, individual personal preferences and factors related to the disease of dementia. Previously some of the behavioural factors were termed antecedents (Aselage and Amella, 2010) indicating that they occurred before declining eating abilities; and although many of the factors that affect behaviour impact on eating abilities a person can still experience declining eating abilities without behavioural symptoms. With such a complex set of interactions happening at a mealtime with eating abilities and meal behaviours often occurring simultaneously, it makes it hard to say for sure if one predicts the other. The importance in the flow of the diagram is that in the end these mealtime abilities have the same consequences for the person living with dementia if no interventions are made.

Factors affecting reduced mealtime abilities

It is important to understand the factors that contribute to a decrease in mealtime abilities and the consequences a reduction in mealtime abilities can cause for the person with dementia; this is shown in Figure 2.1.

As dementia advances, changes to the brain manifest as impairments such as apraxia (a motor disorder caused by damage to the brain), which can affect the ability to eat; agnosia (a neurological disorder resulting in an inability to recognise objects, persons, smells or sounds), which may affect recognition of food or of how a carer is attempting to provide assistance; or dysphagia, which affects the ability to swallow safely (Vitale *et al.*, 2009). Cognitive impairment and physiological changes in dementia result in the reduced ability to eat and drink, which can lead to dysphagia or swallowing difficulties and may prevent assistance from being accepted, contributing to a loss of independence at mealtimes (Chang and Roberts, 2008; Aselage and Amella, 2010; Lin *et al.*, 2010; Lee and Song, 2015). Finally social, cultural and environmental factors contribute to a change in mealtime abilities and especially in behavioural changes (Chang and Roberts, 2008; Lee and Song, 2015). Overall the inability to eat independently means people living with dementia are at an increased risk of malnutrition (Lee and Song, 2015).

Consequences of reduced mealtime abilities

There are many consequences for the person living with dementia if their mealtime abilities continue to decline as highlighted in Figure 2.1. These include an increased risk of inadequate nutritional and fluid intake (Steele *et al.*, 1997; Reed *et al.*, 2005; Lin *et al.*, 2010), leading to dehydration and weight loss (Durnbaugh, Haley and Roberts, 1996; Hanson *et al.*, 2013), which in turn leads to malnutrition, further poor health and decreased quality of life (Smith and Greenwood, 2008; Gilmore-Bykovskyi, 2015).

Typically it is the recorded weight loss rather than the reduction in mealtime abilities that triggers carers and healthcare professionals to intervene. This is often because they are unaware of the changes in mealtime abilities as dementia progresses. This can also call into question reasons for the weight loss, which can be viewed as due to the progression of the disease and therefore considered as a predictor of terminal decline. If the weight loss is mainly due to decreased mealtime abilities and lack of appropriate support then it may be that the weight loss can actually be reversed (Hanson *et al.*, 2013).

The loss of mealtime abilities to eat independently has been shown to be the dominant factor in low food intake, with other main factors including lack of assistance, having unrecognised moderate dependence levels, fewer family visits and having a swallowing difficulty (Reed *et al.*, 2005; Lin *et al.*, 2010). Other general factors include further medical conditions and depression (Lin *et al.*, 2010). In addition 35 per cent had positioning problems at a meal which can be a factor for reduced food and fluid intake (Steele *et al.*, 1997).

There are also consequences for both paid and unpaid carers and healthcare professionals, including increased stress and anxiety and a daunting feeling associated with mealtimes (Watson, 1996; Aselage, 2010; Aselage, Amella and Watson, 2011). Considering that in those with severe dementia up to 88 per cent can receive assistance at mealtimes with more than half requiring full feeding assistance (Steele *et al.*, 1997) the impact on quality of life for both the carer and person with dementia should not be overlooked.

Prevalence of mealtime abilities

How much mealtime abilities in dementia are declining is hard to quantify because of differences in definitions and the ways in which research is carried out. Overall prevalence data suggests that a reduction in mealtime abilities affects 25 per cent to 87 per cent of people living with dementia (see Table 2.1). This table gives an overview of the prevalence rates and the method used to measure this. Often the method involved is a mealtime-abilities assessment tool, and further details on these are provided in Chapter 3 along with a discussion on how to assess mealtime abilities.

Table 2.1: Prevalence of mealtime abilities in people
living with dementia, and method of assessment

Method for measuring prevalence of mealtime abilities (Reference of method study)	Prevalence of reduced mealtime abilities (Reference of prevalence study)
Eating Behaviour Scale (EBS) (Tully et al., 1997)	25% of 98 in long-term care (Wu and Lin, 2015)
Aversive Feeding Behaviours Inventory (AFBI) (Rivière et al., 2002)	27% of 193 living in the community saw a decline in mealtime abilities over one year (Rivière et al., 2002)
Loss of eating ability defined if the person required assistance to put food in the mouth or did not eat at all	41% of 120 in nursing home (Slaughter et al., 2011)
Feeding Abilities Assessment (FAA) (LeClerc et al., 2004)	51% of 153 residents in long-term care (LeClerc et al., 2004)
Survey (unexplained) (Vitale et al., 2009)	58% of 71 residents in a dementia special care unit (Vitale et al., 2009)
Edinburgh Feeding Evaluation in Dementia (EdFED) Scale (Watson, 1996)	60% of 93 people living with dementia in Taiwanese nursing homes (Chang, 2012); 61% of 477 in long-term care (Lin et al., 2010)
Mealtime Assistance Screening Tool (MAST) (Steele et al., 1997)	87% of 349 nursing home residents (Steele et al., 1997)
Feeding Behaviour Inventory (FBI) (Durnbaugh, Haley and Roberts, 1996)	100% of 20 people with Alzheimer's disease (who also ate less than three-quarters of food given to them)
Level of Eating Independence Scale (LEI) (Coyne and Hoskins, 1997)	24 residents in nursing home but no prevalence reported
Structured Meal Observation (SMO) (Reed et al., 2005)	407 residents in long-term care but no prevalence reported

Studies assessing prevalence are mainly confined to people living with dementia in institutional settings, with a lack of data on a free-living population. One study looking at care provided at home reported that over a one-year period mealtime abilities reduced in 27 per cent of people living with dementia at home with their carers (Rivière et al., 2002). As more people with dementia are to be cared for in their own homes, information on the prevalence of mealtime abilities for those being cared for at home will become more important.

One of the earliest prevalence studies using a 'Mealtime Assessment Screening Tool' showed that as many as 87 per cent of 349 residents living with dementia in a care home had at least one 'eating difficulty' (Steele *et al.*, 1997). Out of these, 40 per cent presented with 'challenging behaviour' including drowsiness, interfering body movements, distractibility and hostility. Dysphagia (swallowing difficulties) was also common, being seen in 68 per cent of these 349 care home residents. This was an important study at the time as it clearly showed that there were many factors that had the potential to affect nutritional intake which are not commonly assessed and therefore not treated. It also highlighted that a large percentage of residents with dementia in care homes experienced declining mealtime abilities, and emphasised the complex caring task and resource and training needs required to ensure optimal nutritional intake and maintain quality of life.

Predictors of reduced mealtime abilities

Although the definition of mealtime abilities and how best to measure these is still open for debate, there are at least some very clear findings from research looking at the prevalence and predictors of reduced mealtime abilities.

The vast majority of studies showed that as cognitive abilities declined and dementia becomes more severe, or indeed the longer the duration of dementia, then mealtime abilities also decline (Steele *et al.*, 1997; Berkhout, Cools and Van Houwelingen, 1998; Lin *et al.*, 2010; Slaughter *et al.*, 2011; Chang, 2012; Lee and Song, 2015; Wu and Lin, 2015). In other words the longer you live with dementia or the more rapidly it progresses the higher the chances you have of experiencing a loss of eating abilities and mealtime behaviours. To compound this there is a likely link between rapid cognitive decline and increased undernutrition (Brooke and Ojo, 2015). Therefore if a person with later-stage dementia is not eating well they are likely to have reduced mealtime abilities that will prevent them from increasing their food intake and, as they slowly become malnourished, the severity of dementia continues to increase more rapidly. This at least seems true in long-term care populations (nursing homes, assisted living and residential care) where you would expect those with declining cognitive and physical functioning to reside as they are too complex to be cared for at home.

Several of these same studies however also highlighted that many of the identified mealtime abilities were attributed to causes other than dementia. Greater physical dependence, more comorbidities, less supportive mealtime environments and a lower body mass index (BMI) predicts who was more likely to have reduced mealtime abilities (Berkhout et al., 1998; Slaughter et al., 2011; Chang, 2012).

The final interesting point that is clear from all studies is that this decline in mealtime abilities is observed all around the world, although there is a lack of research including Black and minority ethnic populations. Despite different cultural norms, values and beliefs, eating abilities and behaviours associated with mealtimes are the same worldwide; therefore research and development of successful interventions will benefit everyone (Aselage et al., 2011).

Summary

As dementia progresses and the disease becomes more severe a reduction in mealtime abilities are observed along with a decrease in food and fluid consumption and loss of body weight. It is often not the disease of dementia itself that causes weight loss but changes in eating behaviours and loss of eating abilities (Berkhout et al., 1998). Each person with dementia is different and eating abilities or meal behaviours do not decline along some set defined continuum. However to generalise the observations seen in the research, the most common trend in declining mealtime abilities related to the progression of dementia is provided in Figure 2.2.

Early to mid-stage dementia ─────────────────▶ Later-stage dementia			
Reduced abilities to eat and drink	Changes in preferences and choice of foods	Reduced oral abilities and oral behaviours	Changes in meal behaviours

Figure 2.2: *Generalised overview of the relation between the progression of dementia and eating abilities and behaviours at a mealtime*

Different types of dementia can affect different abilities to eat and drink (Ikeda et al., 2002). Prior to observing a reduction in abilities at a mealtime it may be noticed that someone may forget to eat or forget they have eaten. As indicated in Figure 2.2, when dementia advances past the early stages the most common changes observed first are a reduction in self-feeding abilities. This can include the reduced ability to use cutlery or tableware or finding it hard to recognise a mealtime situation. Typically these changes are often observed alongside changes in the person's preferences for food as taste and smell senses decline and appetite and satiety may decrease. For example, a preference for sweet foods or particular types and textures of foods may be seen alongside not eating the entire meal. These changes often coincide with weight loss and a reduction in food intake. As dementia progresses to a later stage a reduction in oral abilities associated with dysphagia and swallowing difficulties can become more common along with a change in the texture of food consumed (Aselage and Amella, 2010; Aselage et al., 2011). Finally as dementia advances further a person may not be able to communicate their needs through conversation, and a change in meal behaviours is observed. This can lead to irritability or agitation for the individual as the eating abilities that remain are not being supported and their preferences are not being met. This can culminate in increased assistance being provided by carers although commonly this can often increase resistance from the person with dementia. If a person with dementia has reduced mealtime abilities like this then by the time they are in the later stages they can have an accumulation of issues which if not supported will severely affect their ability to maintain their nutrition and hydration.

There are common factors affecting meal behaviours and eating abilities, and health-related outcomes worsen if these mealtime abilities are not supported as shown in Figure 2.1. This often starts with the loss of independence to eat which leads to increased risk of malnutrition and decreased health, wellbeing and quality of life (LeClerc et al., 2004). The progression of dementia to later stages can coincide with reduced mealtime abilities while a decrease in food intake and a loss of weight at the same time could further increase the severity of the dementia symptoms and abilities to eat and drink.

To avoid the loss of independence, early identification of mealtime abilities is required and should be assessed before the need to provide partial or full feeding assistance. Following this assessment, appropriate interventions designed to maintain or enhance mealtime abilities and to provide the most supportive environment must be put in place. This type of approach will improve the chances of maintaining mealtime abilities for as long as possible.

For the carer this can also protect them against the increased burden faced every day at mealtimes when they are required to feed the person with dementia, when in fact they could be using alternative methods to promote independence and self-feeding. Being aware of mealtime abilities and having the knowledge to assess and support these abilities appropriately will be beneficial for the carer as well as the person with dementia.

The next chapter will look at ways to assess mealtime abilities to help plan practical interventions to encourage the preservation of mealtime abilities and independence of people living with dementia at mealtimes.

3

Assessing and Preserving Mealtime Abilities in Dementia

Assessing mealtime abilities

There are many complexities that arise at mealtimes regarding a person living with dementia being able to eat and drink independently, as discussed in the previous chapter and highlighted in Figure 2.1. This highly complex mealtime process means it is very difficult to successfully measure observations at mealtimes owing to the many variables affecting intake.

There are several valid and reliable nutritional assessment tools that are used extensively in healthcare practice and to screen for risk of malnutrition. There is however a paucity of tools that assess mealtime abilities in people with dementia (Aselage, 2010). Nevertheless it is important to do this, not only because they impact on health outcomes and quality of life but also because knowing the level of abilities helps to plan appropriate and effective interventions (Eberhardie, 2004; Aselage, 2010). Currently in health and social care there is no formal approach to assessing mealtime abilities and this needs to change. Helping a person with later-stage dementia to eat independently is a complex task and using a mealtime assessment tool is a consistent way to identify the people who need more support to eat well at mealtimes.

The most valid mealtime assessment tools

From the mid-1990s to the mid-2000s several different mealtime assessment tools were devised and researched. The basis of these tools was to help those caring for someone living with dementia to correctly identify the range of mealtime abilities that can occur. All the tools are observational in nature, which is an appropriate method for assessment of mealtime abilities (Aselage, 2010). This means a carer is required to observe a person with dementia at a mealtime and record their observations on the assessment tool.

More recently the topic of assessing mealtime abilities has been revisited with a new 'Chinese Feeding Difficulty Index' (Ch-FDI) that has been developed and psychometrically tested. The authors felt there were 'no suitable assessment tools available', hence they created a new one (M.F. Liu *et al.*, 2015). Looking at the range of assessment tools available it seems there is much disagreement between researchers on how best to assess mealtime abilities but also about what these tools should be used for. The Ch-FDI once again places an emphasis on feeding the person with dementia, with the tool being designed to be used in assessing those who already require feeding assistance. (However, it should be noted that this is considered normal practice in the culture under investigation where restraint while feeding is common.)

Previous reviews of mealtime assessment tools provide an overview of their validity and reliability (Aselage, 2010). As this book will not dwell on the psychometric analyses used to evaluate validity and reliability it is suggest those interested read the paper mentioned. For clarity of available mealtime assessment tools, however, updated tables from this review paper and further research on mealtime assessment tools will be provided in this chapter. Table 3.1 looks at eight assessment tools used in research and provides a brief overview for each of: its validity and reliability; what healthcare professional it is designed to be used by; how long it takes to administer the tool; what mealtime abilities are assessed; and in what population and setting it was researched.

Table 3.2 provides details on the specific assessments used, whether any interventions are suggested and if the tool has the individual with dementia at the heart of the assessment by providing person-centred aims of care.

Table 3.1: Mealtime assessment tools: validity, healthcare professional use, abilities assessed, length of assessment, population and setting

Assessment tool (reference)	Validity or reliability	Who can use and when and for how long	Mealtime abilities assessed	Diagnoses of dementia and setting
Edinburgh Feeding Evaluation in Dementia (EdFED) Scale (Watson, 1996)	Validity and reliability reported	Dementia care specialist nurses Takes 10–15 minutes to observe one person at one meal	'Aversive feeding behaviours' (meal behaviours related to feeding only)	Moderate to severe dementia in long-term specialist dementia care units (hospital)
Feeding Behavior Inventory (FBI) (Durnbaugh, Haley and Roberts, 1996)	Reliability reported	Geriatric nurse specialists Observation is on one person over one entire mealtime	'Mealtime feeding behaviours' (eating abilities and behaviours)	Mid-stage to moderate Alzheimer's disease in long-term care
Level of Eating Independence Scale (LEI) (Coyne and Hoskins, 1997)	Reliability reported	Nurses Observation is on one person over one entire meal	'Eating behaviours' (eating abilities only)	Dementia (all types) in a long-term care dementia nursing home
Mealtime Assistance Screening Tool (MAST) (Steele et al., 1997)	Not reported	Multidisciplinary team (swallowing team and other specific disciplines) Observation is on one person over one entire meal	'Mealtime difficulties' (eating abilities and behaviours)	Dementia (all types) in long-term care (assisted living, hospital and care home)
Aversive Feeding Behaviours Inventory (AFBI) (Rivière et al., 2002)	Not reported	Not fully reported Assessment was made by research team (but may have included interviewing the carer)	'Aversive feeding behaviours' (eating abilities and behaviours)	Alzheimer's disease in community setting (home care)
Feeding Abilities Assessment (FAA) (LeClerc et al., 2004)	Validity and reliability reported	Assessment was made by research assistants observing one person during their meal (pilot study indicated that it takes five minutes to complete but time of use was not reported in full study)	'Abilities related to feeding affected by ideational apraxia' (eating abilities only)	Dementia (all types) in long-term dementia care facilities

cont.

Assessment tool (reference)	Validity or reliability	Who can use and when and for how long	Mealtime abilities assessed	Diagnoses of dementia and setting
Structured Meal Observation (SMO) (Reed et al., 2005)	Validity and reliability reported	Assessment was made by research team observing up to five residents during one mealtime	'Resident experience during mealtime' (resident need, staff assistance, environmental context and mealtime outcomes rather than specific eating abilities or behaviours)	Dementia (all types) in long-term care (residential care/assisted living and nursing homes)
Eating Behaviour Scale (EBS) originally produced by Tully et al., 1997 (Keller et al., 2006)	Not reported	Dietitians observing residents at mealtimes Termed 'Meal Rounds' Length of observations not reported	'Feeding behaviours' (eating abilities and behaviours)	Dementia (all types) in long-term special dementia care

Table 3.2: Mealtime assessment tools: interventions, assessment and person-centredness

Assessment tool (reference)	Interventions provided as part of the tool	Details on the assessment (items/categories/scoring)	Person-centred?
Edinburgh Feeding Evaluation in Dementia (EdFED) Scale (Watson, 1996)	No	10 questions One category (feeding) Three possible scores for feeding behaviour seen (never = 0, sometimes = 1, often = 2) Higher score indicates more serious feeding behaviours	No. The EdFED only focuses on feeding rather than promoting abilities to reduce dependence on feeding
Feeding Behavior Inventory (FBI) (Durnbaugh, Haley and Roberts, 1996)	No	33-item checklist Four categories (1. resistive/disruptive behaviours, 2. oral behaviours, 3. pattern of intake, 4. style of eating) No scoring but checklist marked dichotomously (seen or not seen)	Potentially but only with a change in language used. The completed FBI helps identify individuals' mealtime abilities but does not suggest how to enhance these abilities

Level of Eating Independence Scale (LEI) (Coyne and Hoskins, 1997)	Yes (verbal prompting and positive reinforcement)	Nine items Two categories (1. eating solid foods, 2. drinking liquids) Four possible scores (total dependence = 1, partial dependence = 2, partial independence = 3, total independence = 4) Lower scores indicate a loss of independence	Yes. Focus of LEI is to improve the level of eating independence but it has a narrow focus on abilities and interventions, limiting its effectiveness
Mealtime Assistance Screening Tool (MAST) (Steele et al., 1997)	No	Checklist format with multiple items Four categories (1. inadequate intake, 2. poor positioning, 3. behavioural impairment, 4. swallowing-related problems (including dentition) Weighted scores for each item with higher scores indicating reduced mealtime abilities	Potentially but only with a change in language used. The MAST provides a thorough assessment of mealtime abilities and other factors affecting nutritional intake but it is staff and time intensive. No interventions are suggested
Aversive Feeding Behaviours Inventory (AFBI) (Rivière et al., 2002)	No	26-item checklist Four categories (1. selective behaviours, 2. resistive behaviours, 3. general dyspraxia, 4. oropharyngeal dysphagia) Scoring not reported	Potentially but only with a change in language used. The AFBI focuses on feeding and does not suggest how to promote abilities to reduce dependence on feeding
Feeding Abilities Assessment (FAA) (LeClerc et al., 2004)	Yes (ranging across verbal cueing, step-by-step verbal instructions, imitation and verbal instructions and finally physical assistance)	32-item checklist Two categories (1. assessment, 2. interventions) No scoring but checklist marked dichotomously ('yes' for a retained ability and 'no' for lost abilities)	Yes. The FAA promotes independence and provides an assessment of eating abilities, and interventions can be designed and targeted to enhance abilities or compensate for lost ones. It does not cover all mealtime abilities commonly observed, so its effectiveness is focused on the ability to self-feed only

cont.

Assessment tool (reference)	Interventions provided as part of the tool	Details on the assessment (items/categories/scoring)	Person-centred?
Structured Meal Observation (SMO) (Reed et al., 2005)	No	28 items reported Categories not fully explained Scoring not reported	A lack of explanation about the SMO means it is difficult to appraise. Is the only tool that provides a short list of environmental considerations but does not link this to how changing the environment can enhance abilities or behaviours
Eating Behaviour Scale (EBS) originally produced by Tully et al., 1997 (Keller et al., 2006)	Yes (verbal prompts and physical assistance)	Six items Three possible scores per item (independent = 3, verbal prompts = 2, dependent = 1) Lower scores indicate a loss of independence	Yes. The focus of the EBS is to promote independence; however, it only assesses six 'feeding behaviours', therefore its use is limited and the interventions used may not accurately assess independence levels

Summary of valid mealtime assessment tools

Most of the mealtime assessment tools are broadly similar and some have undergone psychometric testing for validity and reliability (Watson, 2010). To summarise from Table 3.1, despite several assessment tools being developed there is only one that has gone through the most rigorous psychometric testing and has previously been recognised as a valid and reliable resource (Aselage, 2010). This is the Edinburgh Feeding Evaluation in Dementia (EdFED) Scale (Watson, 1996), which has mainly been used in research settings. Despite this resource being validated since 1996 its application in clinical practice has not materialised. In addition despite the 10-question version of EdFED being widely reported as being valid and reliable (Aselage, 2010) and recommended as a best-practice approach (Stockdell and Amella, 2008) it was actually the six-question EdFED that holds this validity and reliability (Watson, 2010). As the creator of the EdFED himself mentions, 'psychometric testing is never complete; the search for construct validity is infinite' (Watson, 2010, p.1). In these wise words Roger Watson eludes to the fact that tools assessing mealtime abilities will need to be adapted as we understand more about the condition under assessment. Most likely in today's health care, over 20 years on from when the EdFED was originally published, it would not actually achieve construct validity, as the focus of the tool is on the challenges of feeding and does not promote the enhancement of mealtime abilities or reduce dependence on carers (LeClerc *et al.*, 2004). This would in turn affect the EdFED's content validity as it would not be considered to assess all the domains involved in supporting mealtime abilities and other domains including independence, social interactions and choice and preferences (Reimer and Keller, 2009).

The tool also encourages carers to focus on the deficits of the person with dementia and does not provide recommendations for options to support them; therefore it is not considered a person-centred approach. Another point to consider is that the EdFED was developed for and used by experienced nurses working in specialist long-term dementia care who were familiar with the people with dementia they were assessing (Watson, 2010). This important point, which has also been made by the author of the tool, has been neglected in reviews. Nowadays dementia is found in all care settings and all levels of staff will care for people living with dementia, as will family carers. In fact quite often it is not experienced, highly skilled nurses who provide the direct care for people living with dementia but rather healthcare assistants or care staff with very little training or experience. For the majority of staff an assessment tool such as the EdFED will not provide much help as you need a good knowledge of dementia and the person you are caring for to use it appropriately. Perhaps this is one of the main reasons it has not been adapted into routine care. Finally the EdFED only helps recognise 10 main 'feeding difficulties' and does not take into account the environmental and social aspects around a mealtime that could be affecting food intake. Despite the EdFED's psychometric validation in a research setting this does not mean it will be used in a real-life setting without problems. As with many assessment tools, the validity and reliability have been tested but not its practicality for everyday use with a particular client group (Eberhardie, 2004).

The EdFED, despite being a valid resource, probably lacks the practical application to make it useful in the majority of settings and with the majority of carers. There are several other assessment tools that may be useful and more practical (included in Tables 3.1 and 3.2) but they are not psychometrically valid and reliable. However, perhaps this is not important for the carer and there are other ways to ensure a resource is valid and reliable rather than always reverting to the standard scientific psychometric methods. Assessing quality of life or independence or other improved outcomes from using the assessment tool can all provide validity for its use.

Practicalities of mealtime assessment tool options

As the focus of the majority of research on mealtime assessment tools has been based on feeding the person with dementia, it makes choosing an appropriate tool to use in caring and clinical practice difficult.

As detailed in Table 3.1 all but one of the tools have been developed for long-term care settings with their primary use being for research purposes (Aselage, 2010). The majority of tools have been developed by, designed for and used by nurses working in long-term care settings. In modern care nurses are not employed in every setting and healthcare assistants provide much of the mealtime care. Only two tools have utilised the wider range of allied health professionals including a multidisciplinary team (MDT) (MAST) or dietitian-observed assessment (EBS). One tool was used in the community setting (people's own homes) but used research assistants to implement the assessment AFBI. The most effective assessment tool is one that can be used by a number of healthcare professionals (Aselage and Amella, 2012) and perhaps more importantly should also include use by informal carers as they are more likely to provide day-to-day mealtime care.

The tools in general look at assessing both eating abilities and meal behaviours, with two focusing purely on eating abilities (LEI, FAA), one assessment tool measuring 'resident experience during mealtime' (SMO) and one tool focusing on the carer (nurse) providing assistance to feed the person living with dementia (EdFED). Ideally the interest should be focused on the abilities of the person living with dementia and affected by the disease and the environment, rather than the amount of assistance provided by carers (FAA). Carers report that feeding people with dementia is one of the most difficult caring duties (AFBI); therefore energy and care skills should be focused towards enhancing abilities so the person with dementia can continue to feed themselves for as long as possible.

The final column in Table 3.1 highlights what type of dementia the assessment tools have been used for, with most being used in all types of dementia and two focusing on Alzheimer's disease (FBI, AFBI). Not all studies could identify the stage of dementia but considering that nearly all the studies were based in long-term care we can assume most participants were in the later stages. One study identified moderate to severe dementia stages (EdFED) and another mid-to-moderate Alzheimer's disease (FBI).

Referring to Table 3.2 only three out of eight of the assessment tools included interventions a carer can practically implement once the level of mealtime abilities have been identified. All three of these interventions were based on cueing techniques including verbal prompting, positive reinforcement and physical assistance (LEI, EBS, FAA). Assessing the current level of abilities at mealtimes is just the start of the process; the other important aspect is clearly what you do next and this is what the rest of the book will address. Most tools suggest interventions can be planned but provide no practical way of doing this apart from involving healthcare professionals to plan them and create a care plan.

A very positive aspect of the reviewed assessment tools is that the majority can be used as part of a person-centred care approach. Three of the tools are completely focused on improving independence at a mealtime through assessment and structured interventions (LEI, EBS, FAA). Other tools would need to be adapted towards dementia language guidelines as discussed in Chapter 1 so their focus is more centred on abilities rather than difficulties (EdFED, MAST). These tools would also require a range of interventions that promote person-centred approaches to be included as part of the tool.

Finally the major consideration for practical use of a mealtime assessment tool is its availability (Aselage, 2010). One tool is freely available on the internet (EdFED) while the others require access to scientific journals or will need to be adapted or recreated to provide a useable format. No tools are available in an internet-based or electronic form.

The Dementia Mealtime Assessment Tool

In reviewing the available assessment tools it has been commented that the most effective assessment tool is one that can be used by a range of healthcare professionals over a range of settings which is ideally validated (Aselage and Amella, 2012). Considering the disagreement in terms of describing mealtime abilities (Chang and Roberts, 2008) – and the current range of tools available, many of which have not been validated (Aselage, 2010), and new ones continuing to emerge (M.F. Liu *et al.*, 2015) – this is aspirational rather than realistic. It would take many, many years for an assessment tool to be agreed upon and validated across different settings and healthcare professionals. This also neglects the one set of carers providing the majority of care: the unpaid carer at home in the community. What is desirable is a practical tool to support those caring for people with dementia regardless of setting or caring experience. Improving mealtime care starts with assessment; to provide a more practical option for carers a 'Dementia Mealtime Assessment Tool' will be described as a simple way to assess mealtime abilities, and this is used throughout the book (DMAT, 2017). However, any of the assessment tools described in this chapter can be used with awareness of their possible limitations.

The Dementia Mealtime Assessment Tool (DMAT) is an amalgamation of previous research based on the mealtime assessment tools described in Tables 3.1 and 3.2 and using information from further related studies after conducting an extensive literature review. The DMAT is provided in full in Table 3.3. It is a simple tick-box observation-based assessment form which places an emphasis on the identification of common mealtime abilities observed in people living with dementia, providing a structured way to identify these abilities. The DMAT is freely available in a downloadable paper format and can also be accessed as part of an online software system (DMAT, 2017).

The DMAT has not undergone psychometric validation but despite this the tool is seen as a useful addition to the available mealtime care resources available. When comparing a range of mealtime assessment tools the DMAT was the only one that covered all five of the component areas of dementia care under investigation: quality of life, nutrition and hydration, oral and pharyngeal swallow skills, cognition, and environment (Tristani, 2016). The DMAT was highlighted as an easily accessible and useful screening and assessment tool alongside the EdFED and Eating Assessment Tool (EAT-10) (Dutton, 2017).

The four sections of the DMAT as shown in Table 3.3 are designed to help identify reduced mealtime abilities but also (importantly) provide a much-needed structure for carers to be able to adopt person-centred care approaches. A study (Reimer and Keller, 2009) that looked at the past two decades of research literature on mealtime experience and mealtime assistance identified four key person-centred care principles:

1. providing choices and preferences

2. supporting independence

3. showing respect

4. promoting social interactions.

In particular, care principles 1 and 2 strongly overlap with sections 1 and 2 in the DMAT and prompt carers towards person-centred care principles at the mealtime. The interventions discussed later in the book provide the practical means to support all four of these principles.

- Section 1 of the DMAT assesses the 'Ability to self-feed'. By enhancing these abilities you can support the person with dementia to maintain independence and dignity at mealtimes for longer.

- Section 2 assesses 'Preferences and choice with eating and drinking'. This section highlights the person's preferences and needs at a mealtime.

- Section 3 assesses 'Oral abilities and behaviours', which are closely linked to swallowing difficulties. It is very important that appropriate referral to a speech and language therapist for swallowing difficulties is sought if identified and this is further discussed in Chapter 8.

- Section 4 assesses 'meal behaviours', which are often supported by creating a supportive mealtime environment.

The four sections of the DMAT will be used as the basis for the four evidence-based chapters (4, 6, 8 and 10), while Chapters 5, 7, 9 and 11 will provide the practical interventions for supporting the identified mealtime abilities with a person-centred approach.

Table 3.3: The Dementia Mealtime Assessment Tool (DMAT)

	Please tick observed abilities		
Mealtime observations: **Ability to self-feed**	Not seen	Seen once	Seen repeatedly
Reduced ability to use cutlery (spoon, fork or knife)			
Reduced ability to get food onto cutlery (spoon, fork or knife)			
Reduced ability to cut meat (or other foods)			
Reduced ability in identifying food from plate			
Plate slides or is moved around the table			
Reduced ability using cups or glasses			
Reduced ability seeing or identifying cups or glasses			
Spills drinks when drinking			
Stares at food without eating			
Falls asleep or is asleep during mealtime			
Mealtime observations: **Preferences with eating and drinking**	Not seen	Seen once	Seen repeatedly
Prefers sweet food or eats desserts/sweets first			
Only eats certain foods			
Eats (or drinks) too fast			
Mixes food together			
Does not eat lunch but eats breakfast and some dinner			
Eats very small amounts of food (or drink)			
Slow eating or prolonged mealtimes			
Mealtime observations: **Oral abilities and behaviours**	Not seen	Seen once	Seen repeatedly
Bites on cutlery (spoon, fork, knife)			
Does not open mouth			
Holds food or leaves food in mouth			
Spits out food			
Reduced ability chewing			
Prolonged chewing without swallowing			
Does not chew food before swallowing			
Reduced ability swallowing or refusing to swallow			

Mealtime observations: Meal behaviours	Not seen	Seen once	Seen repeatedly
Hoards, hides, throws or plays with food			
Eats other people's food (or drink)			
Refuses to eat (verbally or physically)			
Bats away or pushes away spoon presented by carer			
Turns head away when being fed			
Distracted from eating			
Demonstrates impatient behaviour around mealtimes			
Eats small amounts and leaves table			
Walks during mealtime or unable to sit still for meals			
Shows agitated behaviour or irritability			

Key:
    Not seen = mealtime ability maintained
    Seen once = reduced mealtime ability observed at least once
    Seen repeatedly = reduced mealtime ability observed twice or more often

Preserving mealtime abilities

Due to the complexities of providing nutritional care at mealtimes, a structured assessment, intervention and monitoring cycle, with the person with dementia at the heart of it, is key to maintaining person-centred care but also for improving outcomes. Figure 3.1 identifies a continuous mealtime care cycle which involves five phases to help develop a person-centred approach, achieve positive changes to mealtime care and hopefully improve health outcomes. Structured approaches such as this are not new in health and social care but unfortunately are not always implemented effectively. In dementia care the most recognised structured approach for developing person-centred practice and achieving practice change is the Dementia Care Mapping cycle (University of Bradford, 2017).

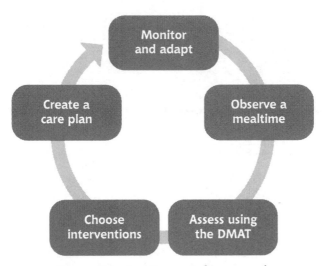

Figure 3.1: *A continuous mealtime care cycle*

Observe a mealtime

The person with dementia being assessed at the mealtime will be observed by their carer when they consume their main meal. It is best to observe the main meal as this will require the most cognitive skills to successfully consume the food; for example if you are observing someone eating a sandwich then they will not be using a knife and fork. Similarly by observing someone eating soup or cereal they are only using a spoon so the task is not as complex. The only exception to this rule is if you care for someone who only eats sandwiches and soups, as this is as complex as their eating becomes. Mealtime abilities can fluctuate throughout the day and from day to day (Young and Greenwood, 2001) owing to factors such as fatigue and environment; therefore it may be appropriate to assess at different mealtimes depending on the individual.

The observer (the carer) will witness the person living with dementia from a distance far enough to see everything they do but not too close as to interfere or feel like they are intruding on the person's mealtime.

Assess using the DMAT

While observing, the carer will record all mealtime observations on the DMAT utilising a simple tick-box assessment. It should take roughly seven to ten minutes to complete the DMAT on each person observed at a mealtime. It is possible to observe two people or more at once in an acute (hospital) or institutionalised (e.g. care home) setting, for example on a hospital ward or in a dining room.

Choose interventions

Assessment of mealtime abilities is an essential first step to recognising the current level of independence but the true value of assessment comes from formulating an effective person-centred care plan. Resources are needed to help carers find the link between specific changes in mealtime abilities and effective interventions (Aselage, 2010). The following chapters will concentrate on providing the missing link between assessment and interventions related to mealtime abilities and improving nutrition and hydration. Tips on choosing suitable interventions and not making the interventions themselves too complex are also discussed.

Create a care plan

Using the information gained from the mealtime assessment and the suggested interventions chosen, a care plan specific to the person's needs can be produced and shared among carers. It is important to record what specific mealtime abilities are reduced and what interventions are to be trialled to support these abilities.

Monitor and adapt

The overall aims of this process are:

1. to help the carer to be better equipped to identify the current level of mealtime abilities and then (most importantly) using the suggested interventions, enhance these abilities through a person-centred care plan

2. to improve a range of health outcomes for the person with dementia, for example improved food intake, enhanced independence, improved eating and drinking abilities or meal behaviours, more appropriate choice of foods, increased body weight and improved quality of life.

A range of monitoring tools may be required to identify the health outcomes listed above.

To measure if the suggested interventions detailed in a care plan have helped support the identified mealtime abilities you again use the DMAT during a mealtime and compare the results obtained to the original observation. It is recommended to complete the DMAT at monthly intervals for the person with dementia to ensure their mealtime abilities are continually assessed and the interventions are adapted as required. If the mealtime abilities have improved then a change in the amount of times the ability is observed will be seen; or if the ability is now retained it will no longer be observed. It may take time for some interventions to show any effect, especially if it requires the person with dementia to become accustomed with a change, for example using adapted cutlery.

Summary

There is a considerable need for better mealtime assessment of people living with dementia in order to identify successful interventions that enhance mealtime abilities and support the person to maintain their independence at mealtimes. There are many tools that assess mealtime abilities which have been available for years and yet have not been used in standard care.

Improving mealtime care starts with improved assessment, and until changes in assessment practices are implemented then the same care will continue to be provided. Typically this means carers reverting to the same old way of doing things with a reliance on feeding the person when they have reduced intake and are losing weight. There are, however, better and more person-centred ways to achieve improved mealtime care.

This chapter proposes an accessible and easy-to-use Dementia Mealtime Assessment Tool and mealtime care cycle to aid those caring for people with dementia at mealtimes. Using a structured approach to assessment and mealtime care and utilising these resources are the first steps towards improved mealtime care practices and person-centred mealtime care.

4

Independence and Dignity at Mealtimes

THE ABILITY TO EAT AND DRINK

Introduction

Eating is one of life's pleasures and the ability to continue feeding oneself as dementia advances is central to feelings of self-control, independence and self-worth. For people with advancing dementia what should be a pleasurable mealtime can too often become a frustrating and exhausting experience if individual needs are not supported in the right way. We learn how to feed ourselves before we learn to talk, walk or even control our bowel movements. This may be one of the reasons why this ability is one of the last activities of daily living we lose (Chang and Roberts, 2008). It is important to note that a correlation exists between the ability to self-feed and losing weight (see Figure 4.1). A study published in 1998 (Berkhout *et al.*, 1998) found that reduced self-feeding abilities and independence at mealtimes led to increased weight loss. However, when eating abilities were improved an increased body weight was seen.

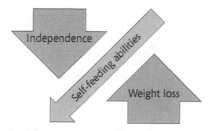

Figure 4.1: *The ability to continue to feed yourself as dementia advances is critical if independence at mealtimes and body weight are to be maintained*

Independence at mealtimes

A loss of eating and drinking abilities means you become dependent on others therefore decreasing independence. For people with dementia this often means being fed at all mealtimes by a carer. For some this assistance is crucial to maintaining adequate nutritional intake; for many others, however, the feeding assistance provided may not be necessary and may in fact harbour increased dependence on being fed as more eating and drinking abilities are reduced (Osborn and Marshall, 1993). By using mealtime assessment methods to first identify eating and drinking abilities and then by implementing supportive interventions, self-feeding abilities can be maintained or regained (W. Liu *et al.*, 2015). Maintaining independence at mealtimes by feeding yourself is therefore extremely important in achieving adequate nutrition and hydration, preventing weight loss and malnutrition, but also to have a positive impact on a person's quality of life while preserving dignity.

Eating and drinking abilities at mealtimes are not commonly assessed, which is often why those identified as struggling to eat and drink are usually provided with feeding assistance. The theory is of course that if you provide more staff to feed people at mealtimes then they will increase their food and fluid intake. Unfortunately this theory is not always proved to be correct in practice. Not everyone with dementia will respond in a positive way to being fed even if high-quality feeding assistance is provided (Simmons, Osterweil and Schnelle, 2001). Whether or not anyone with dementia actually enjoys being fed is debatable; after all most people would certainly prefer to feed themselves at least some of the time. Importantly when feeding someone with dementia, if this does still not improve their food intake then alternative methods must be employed. Carers can waste lots of time and effort trying to feed someone who actually may benefit from other less invasive and less staff-intensive interventions. Carers may actually find that using the interventions described in this chapter can increase eating abilities so those who previously were being fed are able to feed themselves. Discovering what works best for the individual is what person-centred care promotes, and using the assessment and intervention methods described throughout the practical chapters of this book will aid in achieving person-centred care.

Self-feeding abilities

This first of four practical chapters focuses on eating and drinking abilities and in particular the ability to self-feed. Self-feeding abilities are often observed to decline in people living with dementia if they are not supported (Durnbaugh *et al.*, 1996; Coyne and Hoskins, 1997).

Provided below is a list of common eating and drinking abilities that have been shown to be reduced in people living with dementia. This list is reproduced from section 1 of the DMAT discussed in Chapter 3. These particular eating abilities are required to physically get food from the plate to the mouth and therefore they focus on abilities needed to use cutlery and other tableware. Additionally the ability to recognise food and drink is also apparent and is often impacted by loss of vision or visual changes.

Common self-feeding abilities that can affect food and fluid intake

- Reduced ability to use cutlery (spoon, fork or knife)

- Reduced ability to get food onto cutlery (spoon, fork or knife)

- Reduced ability to cut meat (or other foods)

- Reduced ability in identifying food from plate

- Plate slides or is moved around the table

- Reduced ability using cups or glasses

- Reduced ability seeing or identifying cups or glasses

- Spills drinks when drinking

- Stares at food without eating

- Falls asleep or is asleep during mealtime

Adapted from Durnbaugh *et al.* (1996);
Watson (1996); Crawley and Hocking (2011)

There are two important points to consider. First, the abilities related to self-feeding are often the first eating abilities observed to decline in mild to moderate stages of dementia and are also the most common. Those with severe dementia will frequently have other reduced mealtime abilities and meal behaviours in addition to fewer self-feeding abilities, which impact on their nutritional intake and independence. Second, enhancing these abilities may prevent further reductions in eating and drinking abilities. The next section in this chapter will look at the research evidence behind the interventions used to enhance eating and drinking abilities.

The evidence for enhancing self-feeding abilities

The goal of care for enhancing self-feeding abilities at mealtimes is simply to support the person with dementia do as much for themselves for as long as they can. This will extend their independence at mealtimes and help promote their dignity. It will also reduce the need for being fed until completely necessary or with as little assistance from their carer as is required.

The interventions used to achieve this tend to follow a process of care as shown in Figure 4.2 which starts with cueing and encouragement and then involves modifying the table setting and/or tableware. Interventions could also involve the adaptation of food such as providing finger foods, and finally advance with increasing physical and feeding assistance and referral to health professionals for further advice. As a carer follows this process it may start as single interventions, for example verbally prompting the person to eat, but typically filter into a range of multicomponent interventions all designed to support eating and drinking abilities. As the type or number of interventions increases then so does the complexity. This is not to say cueing and encouraging a person with dementia to eat is easy; rather that cueing a person to eat who is using modified cutlery and plates and ensuring the correct nutritional content of finger food, while supporting their abilities with some physical assistance, is yet more complicated. Interventions required will not always follow this process and of course you will need to pick and choose the best approaches based on assessment and monitoring as discussed in Chapter 3.

It is worth noting that the vast majority of research has been carried out in care home settings; however, the suggested interventions for enhancing eating and drinking abilities are applicable to all other care settings.

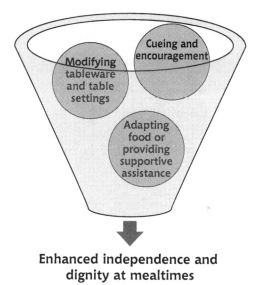

Enhanced independence and dignity at mealtimes

Figure 4.2: *The mealtime intervention mix: supporting eating and drinking abilities*

Providing cueing

Cueing is a term that describes providing a reminder or hint to do something, or to get someone 'back on track', which is why it is often related to orientation. Cueing is something carers do all the time yet limited evaluation of effectiveness has been produced in the research literature. Cueing can also be a common form of interaction between the carer and the person with dementia at a mealtime, and this interaction is important. It has been indicated that the quality of this interaction can affect the amount of food consumed, in that the more positive the interaction, the more is eaten (Aselage *et al.*, 2011). Carers' beliefs around their attitude and approach to providing mealtime assistance can also have an impact. One author described two sets of carers: 1. the 'social feeder' who believed mealtimes were an opportunity to socialise and meet the psychosocial needs of the individuals, and 2. the 'technical feeder' who believed in providing adequate nutrition in a more task-orientated way (Pelletier, 2005).

It is important to know what beliefs the carer holds, as the evidence seems to indicate a balance between the two is needed. The appropriate training and implementation of cueing techniques could then be targeted to the right carer. The aim when cueing is to provide a graduated prompting protocol centred on the person's current ability level so that only the required amount of assistance is provided. This protocol starts with verbal prompts and encouragement, then moves on to manual and physical prompting and finally involves using hand feeding techniques and (if eventually required) full feeding assistance. A mix of these cueing techniques can be used to provide optimal mealtime cueing assistance that enhances self-feeding abilities and increases social interaction throughout the mealtime experience (Simmons *et al.*, 2001). Each one of these will now be discussed.

Verbal prompts

Providing verbal prompts is a simple way to cue a person with dementia at a mealtime. In care homes half the residents with dementia can have reduced eating abilities, and in one study the majority (72%) of these required verbal prompts/cueing or physical assistance to initiate self-feeding (LeClerc *et al.*, 2004). Eating can be improved when carers provide verbal prompts and 'positive reinforcement', which is another phrase for encouragement. In care practice and in research a range of verbal prompts are typically used including direct prompts such as *'Pick up the (name of cutlery)'* or *'Swallow the food'*, while verbal reinforcement can include *'That's right'* or *'Good'* (Coyne and Hoskins, 1997).

How the technique of providing verbal prompts was initiated in one study is described here as an example of a verbal cueing protocol, although in a non-research real-life setting such a structured protocol is of course not necessary. When providing assistance at a mealtime, if the person did not take a bite of food within 15 seconds of being served the meal a verbal cue was provided. Verbal cues were provided throughout the meal if a bite of food was not taken for 15 consecutive seconds. If the person did not respond after three consecutive verbal cues then assistance was stopped for five minutes and then restarted as per the research protocol (Cleary, Hopper and Van Soest, 2012). In reality a carer may initiate some manual prompts at this point. Specific cues to encourage eating along with neutral and positive cues were all used with some examples of these listed here:

Specific cues said by carers:
Have another bite, *or*, take another bite.
How about another bite of your... (*specific food item*)?

Neutral comments said by carers:
The food looks good today.
You seem... (*happy, sad, etc.*) today.

Positive reinforcing comments used by carers:
That's nice, (*name*); now you're eating some of your... (*kind of food*).
You're doing well using your spoon today.

As shown above, the communication used when cueing should be simple, as understanding verbal language can decline as cognition declines. You may notice that those whose first language is not English speak using their traditional language more frequently. Learning some simple phrases for use at the mealtime may be beneficial here.

A commonly reduced eating ability is the 'Reduced ability to use cutlery (spoon, fork or knife)'. This ability can be cued by reminding the person to *'Pick up the fork'* or *'Hold the handle of the spoon in your hand.'* Or when cueing for certain foods or eating practices, other examples of direct specific cueing using closed-ended phrases may include *'Mr Smith, pick up your milk'* or *'Mrs Jones, scoop your peas,'* or *'Swallow please.'* An example of an indirect specific cue using an open phrase may be *'Would you like another bite of chicken?'*

Some general verbal prompting recommendations include the following, adapted from National Food Service Management Institute (2005a, 2005b):

- Appropriately address the person, Mr Smith or George, for example.

- Use brief, simple instructions as above to talk the person through each mealtime step as required.

- Repeat the verbal prompts at each mealtime if required.

- Speak in calm, soothing tones.

- Remember your facial expression; a smile is better than a frown. Other non-verbal interactions include providing eye contact.

- Be patient and do not expect immediate results. You may need to restate or slightly rephrase the verbal prompt. Time invested at this stage may save time later on and the benefits to the person are worth the effort.

- Provide encouragement.

Encouragement

Encouragement, also termed positive reinforcement, is a mainstay of any caring role and is often used in conjunction with cueing. Examples include *'Well done'* or *'That's it, Mr Smith.'* Despite the ease of using positive encouragement it has been observed in only 8 per cent of all verbal interactions at a mealtime. Encouragement can also include gentle coaxing or persuasion, representing 48 per cent of all verbal interactions used at a mealtime (Ullrich and McCutcheon, 2008). Examples of these phrases often observed in this research study were *'Will you have another sip of your drink?'*, *'One more mouthful'* or *'You can do it.'*

In a care home those individuals who eat in their own rooms may not receive as much encouragement as those in the main dining room, as they can be left to their own devices. Often the amount of food eaten is only seen when their food is collected, since carers may not have the time or capacity to encourage individuals outside of the dining room. If this is the case then effort must be made to better engage with these individuals.

Manual prompts

Another form of cueing is providing manual prompts. Prompting someone manually may trigger them to initiate the eating skill. In the example of 'Reduced ability to use cutlery (spoon, fork or knife)' the manual prompt would be to place the fork in the person's hand. Modelling is also a form of a manual prompt and provides a visual cue to the person with dementia that they can imitate. It will help them observe the eating skill, which may help them copy your movements or prompt them to initiate the movement themselves, for example 'modelling' the process of picking up and using your cutlery. Actually eating your meal with someone can also act as a manual prompt and may help support their eating abilities by allowing them to 'follow your lead'. There may be many other benefits too of eating your meals alongside someone and this is discussed in Chapter 6. Unfortunately the use of gesturing or demonstrating eating skills can be observed less often or indeed not at all in dementia care, as carers can place more emphasis on correct positioning of protective clothing and wiping away food spillages (Ullrich and McCutcheon, 2008).

Using verbal cues at the same time as manual cues (to reinforce the eating abilities required) and offering encouragement can also be effective. Remember that progress may be slow but the ultimate aim of preserving dignity and self-worth for the individual is only achieved with increased independence and enhanced eating abilities (National Food Service Management Institute, 2005b).

Finally if caring in a group setting such as a care home, day centre or supportive living where people with dementia eat together, it is worth considering seating arrangements to optimise socialisation. Sit the person with a friend or someone they have an affinity with to enhance social interaction, since this may provide the manual cueing required to support eating abilities. Or if you are already doing this sit them with those who have maintained eating abilities as this may help them continue to feed themselves by taking cues from others. This element of socialisation and social compatibility and its effect on intake at mealtimes is discussed further in Chapter 10.

Reminiscence therapy

Reminiscence therapy at mealtimes involves the use of conversations based on principles of reminiscence in which someone's meaningful past life experiences are discussed. It is argued that using conversation rather than cueing, which tends to be more task focused, provides a more dignified intervention approach to enhance engagement at the mealtime and improve food intake. Practically for the carer this means discovering topics of interest to the person concerned, usually by discussion with them and their family. In one study a scripted reminiscence conversation was used involving a scripted introduction and five talking points based on information provided when speaking to the family members. Or if this was not possible, generic topics were used, for example the weather, activities, pets and so on. The following is an example of a script used in the research (Cleary et al., 2012):

Script #1 – Topic: Farming
Introduction:
I hear that you used to live on a farm.

Question:
Did you enjoy living on a farm?

Comment:
I used to live on a farm, and I really liked it.

Question:
Did you raise cows or did you have crops?

Comment:
We had cows on our farm. Living on a farm is hard work.

The carer would introduce a topic while providing assistance at the mealtime and wait up to 15 seconds for an answer. If no response to the topic was made, it would be repeated, and if this happened for three times a new topic would be introduced. If there was still no response after trying two different topics the reminiscence conversation was ended. If an answer was made then the carer would respond with a comment and continue to introduce topics from the script. The results of the study indicated that using reminiscence therapy was just as effective when compared to verbal cueing. Unfortunately the authors did not combine the verbal cueing with reminiscence therapy to see if this combination was more effective than when used in isolation. What may prevent the common use of reminiscence therapy is the time it takes to implement the technique in practice, which again the authors did not comment on or measure.

The use of reminiscence therapy is consistent with a person-centred approach and provides carers with a way to engage in meaningful and culturally appropriate conversations. It may be that this approach used in combination with other cueing techniques described in this section provides the most beneficial outcomes in terms of both increased social engagement and improved nutritional intake. Finally, a word of caution for those individuals with a swallowing difficulty: it must be ensured that they do not talk with food or fluid in their mouth. The airway may be open during speech when attempting a swallow therefore increasing risk of food or fluid entering the airway (Griffin *et al.*, 2009).

Expressive acts

A final way of cueing and encouragement involves a more expressive act such as gently touching the forearm or gently rubbing the top of the person's hand to get their attention. This type of expressive act is seen less commonly in care at mealtimes (Ullrich and McCutcheon, 2008) but can be another useful caring technique to help orientate the individual to the meal. The use of touch and encouragement to promote communication and comfort may impact food intake and support reduced mealtime abilities (Lin *et al.*, 2010).

Hand feeding techniques

There are three main hand feeding techniques used in the care of people with dementia: the direct hand, hand over hand, and hand under hand (Batchelor-Murphy *et al.*, 2015b). All three techniques take roughly the same amount of time to provide assistance (Batchelor-Murphy *et al.*, 2017). Direct hand is basically as it sounds; it provides full assistance for feeding and should be reserved only for those who are fully dependent on care, but unfortunately it is commonly used the majority of the time (Batchelor-Murphy *et al.*, 2015b). The other two techniques can serve as prompts for the person to feed themselves, unless they have particular physical problems or weakness. By providing a limited amount of assistance using these two techniques, self-feeding abilities can be preserved and promote a better sense of independence. Supporting the individual using hand-under-hand feeding can provide the same amount of food intake as direct feeding and takes no longer to accomplish. Hand-under-hand feeding when compared to hand-over-hand feeding can also reduce other meal behaviours that may affect intake. This is because the hand-under-hand-technique may elicit a sense of control over the eating movement and feel more like the person with dementia has initiated the movement. The hand-over-hand technique may be more appropriate for people who have maintained finer motor control – they can hold cutlery – and is used to guide the cutlery to the mouth. Although hand-under-hand feeding was more effective in one study (Batchelor-Murphy *et al.*, 2016) there is a lack of evidence on feeding techniques, so use the one which seems most accepted by the person you are helping. It is indeed rather troubling that an activity such as hand feeding, which impacts on a person's quality of life, has extremely little evidence detailing when or how to use these techniques as dementia progresses (Batchelor-Murphy *et al.*, 2015b).

Summary of hand feeding techniques:

- Direct hand feeding: reserve only for those fully dependent on care.

- Hand over hand: this may increase meal behaviours.

- Hand under hand: this is the preferred choice when providing feeding assistance.

Summary of cueing

Providing mealtime assistance using cueing (verbal and manual prompts, positive reinforcement, appropriate praise and encouragement) can be effective in improving eating abilities (W. Liu *et al.*, 2015). Unfortunately these interventions are often overlooked when demands on carers' time is high (Vitale *et al.*, 2009). Cueing a person is simply a way of prompting them, while providing encouragement helps reinforce the cueing. The limited research indicates that cueing techniques can improve meal behaviours, increase the amount of food and fluid consumed and help maintain or increase weight, and that they can be combined with other interventions such as increased socialisation through sharing meals to improve participation and communication at mealtimes (Cleary *et al.*, 2012). Evidence suggests that a minimum of one and a maximum of eight cueing interactions, between one and five coaxing interactions and between one and twelve encouragement interactions and interventions are provided at mealtimes by carers per person (Ullrich and McCutcheon, 2008). The amount and type of cueing required will be determined by the needs of the individual and should be assessed and intervened upon in a person-centred way; what works for one person may not work for another. If one cueing technique does not work try another one, or try a combination of techniques until you find the best way to support the person. To achieve this, assessment and monitoring of appropriate interventions are key and resources such as the DMAT can be useful in doing this. A further useful assessment tool specific to using cutlery and providing cueing can be found in the paper by Chantele LeClerc and colleagues (2004). Their 'Feeding Abilities Assessment' tool systematically assesses the ability to use cutlery in both simple and complex tasks and may provide a structured way to record and monitor cueing interventions used to enhance these particular eating abilities.

Providing different forms of cueing can be a long and slow process and both time and patience are required. At times the carer may want to simply stop trying and just start feeding the person, as this is quicker and easier for them. This practice has been and is still very common in dementia care but will likely increase the assistance that is required. Research indicates that institutional practices such as feeding foster dependence and reduce functional abilities to eat (Osborn and Marshall, 1993). When people with dementia are provided with more assistance than they actually need, they lose their ability to respond to cues. They then become more dependent on the carer to provide full feeding assistance, eventually at every meal. The mealtime goals of care therefore should always be driven towards finding interventions that support remaining eating and drinking abilities for as long as possible.

Providing full assistance

Continuous full feeding assistance can be the most common form of physical assistance (47%) in the care of older people with dementia when compared to more sporadic assistance (2%), hand feeding techniques (14%) or manual prompting (33%) (Ullrich and McCutcheon, 2008). More use of these last two cueing interventions must be promoted; however, at some point it may be necessary to provide full assistance as dementia advances to a stage that prevents the person from feeding themselves, no matter what interventions or support are put in place. Before full assistance is implemented it is important to have worked through the cueing interventions discussed previously and only provide full feeding assistance when someone has lost abilities to self-feed.

A study specifically looking at increasing assistance at mealtimes, using all cueing techniques (increased frequency of using verbal, manual and physical prompts) and providing feeding assistance to increase food intake, found this did not work in all participants (Simmons *et al.*, 2001). Half of the people with dementia significantly increased their food and fluid intake during the mealtime but it was ineffective in others. Importantly from a practical perspective the time required of carers to implement the increased assistance greatly exceeded the usual time carers spent assisting at mealtimes, from an average of 9 to 38 minutes per person per meal. This means that although a significant increase in nutrition was achieved the intervention itself is perhaps impractical in standard care. Due to the time-intensive nature of the required assistance and the fact that it only worked in half the people, the authors describe a screening process to help identify who this intensive intervention would be most successful for. This screening process could be invaluable both to the carer and the person with dementia and so is described here.

Screening

When screening for the effectiveness of increased assistance at mealtimes one screening process suggests that an increased level of assistance is provided over a two-day trial to determine effectiveness of any continued assistance. If someone does not increase their food intake during the two days then they are unlikely to, even if more days of assistance are provided. If the increased feeding assistance is effective in increasing intake then this should be continued with those individuals.

To reduce the time required for one-to-one assistance, then, continued assistance for these responsive individuals in a small group of three was shown to still be effective in increasing intake (Simmons et al., 2001). It is worth noting however that a small percentage of people who responded to one-to-one assistance did not respond in the small-group environment, so continued monitoring is still very important if this change is made. This provides a practical way to reduce the time spent by carers assisting at mealtimes while still providing an effective intervention.

It was also found that those with advancing dementia responded better to the increased assistance by eating more while those who were slow eaters responded less well. The authors nonetheless state that the best way to identify who will respond optimally to increased assistance is a one- to two-day trial as mentioned above, rather than relying on the characteristics they displayed.

We often hear that more staff are needed at mealtimes to 'feed' people with dementia. The moral of the story here is that providing more and more staff at mealtimes does not necessarily mean this will increase food and fluid intake as many may be unresponsive to increased one-to-one assistance. If half the people with dementia did not improve their food intake then even when a care home employed twice as many staff at mealtimes intake would still not increase. This is very important and these unresponsive individuals must be correctly identified. Other interventions should be trialled for them, perhaps by improving their own self-feeding abilities through modifying the tableware, cutlery and environment or including more social-based interventions as described later in this chapter and in subsequent chapters. This is only one study and to extrapolate these isolated findings to everyone is unwise; however, it does provide a practical and structured way of identifying which individuals may respond best to full feeding assistance.

Factors to consider

There are some other factors to consider in those who may require feeding assistance. It can be the case that those who require assistance to eat are left till last as those who eat independently are served their meal, and food is cleared from those who finish their meals quickly. One study indicated that residents who require feeding assistance can wait for up to 31 minutes before receiving assistance (Steele *et al.*, 2007). This lengthy wait could impact on their intake owing to overstimulation in an unsupportive mealtime environment, loss of interest in food or becoming tired. The delay in feeding makes sense from the organisation's perspective but is not in the best interest of the person with dementia. If additional staff are required to help these residents then that is what should happen first; leaving the most vulnerable to last should not be considered standard practice.

Mealtime assistance

As mealtime abilities are reduced the general intervention is for carers to provide increased assistance with feeding, leading to a decrease in mealtime independence for the person with dementia. For those with severe dementia up to 88 per cent can receive assistance at mealtimes with more than half requiring full feeding assistance, in other words receiving all their food from being fed by a carer. This percentage can drop to between 30 and 60 per cent of those with moderate cognitive impairment while those without any cognitive impairment (14%) can still require assistance at mealtimes, mainly with help setting up their tray and navigating hard-to-open packaging (Steele *et al.*, 1997).

This increase in feeding assistance can either help with an increase in nutrition or have no significant impact upon food and fluid intake. In one study in nursing homes where assistance was provided, residents with dementia still lost weight despite increased assistance and feeding (Berkhout *et al.*, 1998). This is not always the case; in fact in two studies people experiencing severe dementia and loss of mealtime abilities had better oral intake when receiving full feeding assistance than those who had mild to moderate cognitive impairment and received no assistance (Steele *et al.*, 1997; Wu and Lin, 2015). Carers often experience difficulties providing mealtime assistance and feeding (Chang and Roberts, 2008) which may account for differences in these studies. Several authors (Steele *et al.*, 1997; Lin *et al.*, 2010) have highlighted that the group receiving feeding assistance had at one point likely passed through a stage without receiving any mealtime interventions. This may have led to an increased loss of mealtime abilities and therefore increased dependence on feeding assistance. If priority had been given to assessing a decline in eating abilities in the moderate cognitive-impairment group then interventions could have been put in place. These interventions could help facilitate independence at mealtimes, prevent decreased food intake, enhance the person's wellbeing and limit the need for full feeding assistance.

Summary of full assistance
Before the final stage of providing full feeding assistance is reached, it is important to assess and monitor the effectiveness of the mealtime assistance provided. By using better assessment methods to identify eating and drinking abilities, or screening methods to determine effectiveness of feeding assistance, the needs of these individuals may be met in other ways. Following assessment the carer may find that some people can actually feed themselves, or at least start feeding themselves and get help when needed. Additionally when increased assistance is first introduced close monitoring of food and fluid intake at mealtimes over one to two days should be implemented. This will help determine whether the increase in assistance provided actually equals an increase in nutritional intake.

Modifying the table setting
In the next section the importance of modifying tableware to support the abilities of a person with dementia is discussed along with several research studies looking at the effectiveness of these interventions. Before modifying the actual tableware however, one can simply try modifying the table setting.

This can involve reducing the number of items and cutlery available to choose from, for example simply providing a fork and a meal cut into suitable pieces and removing any other non-eating items, such as salt and pepper pots. Reducing the complexity of the task could be enough to help support some people with dementia to maintain their eating abilities. Combining a simplified table setting with adapted cutlery or modified tableware is usually the next step if abilities still require support.

Modifying tableware

Modifying cutlery and tableware is traditionally seen as an environmental change to the dining environment. As many self-feeding abilities can be preserved or improved by these modifications they are discussed in this chapter, and further changes to the dining environment are discussed in Chapter 10.

Tableware and colour contrast

'We eat with our eyes' is a fantastic and very true expression but unfortunately declining vision with age and the progression of dementia can both affect this natural visual sense. If you are having trouble working out if what has been put in front of you is a plate of food or not, or if it is food that you cannot recognise, then you will probably be less inclined to start eating it.

A range of visual problems have been identified in people diagnosed with dementia of the Alzheimer's type, including loss of visual acuity, colour vision, visual fields and contrast sensitivity along with changes in complex visual functions such as reading and in the naming and identification of objects (Armstrong, 2009). The ability to perceive colour contrast can be exacerbated if older people have dementia and/or glaucoma or cataracts (Brush and Calkins, 2008) as thickening and yellowing of the lens alters the way colour is perceived (Brush, 2001). This means for example that white plates and silver cutlery on a white tablecloth will be harder to visualise as there is hardly any colour contrast between these objects. This can make it difficult to identify the plate from the tablecloth, while the cutlery may seem to blend into the table – making it harder to spot. With dementia there is also an impairment in judging depth perception and spatial orientation (Brush and Calkins, 2008; Timlin and Rysenbry,

2010) due to a decrease in pupil size and reaction time and a loss of elasticity of the lens (Brush, 2001). Dining objects may appear on top of each other, or the edges of objects may be harder to see, or different foods may appear a similar colour and blend into each other. Finding it harder to see the plates, cutlery, fluid in cups or food on the plate can all be affected by a lack of visual contrast. Providing a high visual contrast therefore is a way of cueing the person with dementia to focus on the table setting and meal in front of them.

Limited evidence suggests that people living with dementia can distinguish some colours better than others; however, research of this kind involved looking at coloured paper not coloured plates or table settings. It also did not involve those with reduced eating abilities and may therefore not be relevant (Calkins, 2010). Comparisons between using white vs red tableware found the high-contrast red tableware increased food intake by 25 per cent (Dunne *et al.*, 2004). This often-quoted study, which only included nine participants, is perhaps unfortunately partly to blame for the ghastly red plastic plates available to 'help' people with dementia eat. These plates often look childish and do not provide an attractive presentation when food is placed on them. These brightly coloured plates may also add to the sense of stigma in those made to use them, as their tableware feels vastly different from standard tableware, a point made by Timlin and Rysenbry in their publication *Design for Dementia* (2010). It is unlikely the individual colour of a plate is going to make someone eat more, and more importantly the focus should be on the contrast between colours aiming for a high contrast. There is nothing wrong with a white plate if the food on the plate is bright and colourful, for example pasta covered with tomato sauce, basil leaves and slices of mozzarella, which provides a high contrast between the white plate and predominantly red food. If the meal on a white plate is a plain chicken breast, mashed potato and sweetcorn then the contrast in colours is low as they all look white. In this situation a coloured plate would be a better option as it provides a high contrast between the coloured plate and mainly white food. A dark navy colour can be a good choice as it does not distract from the appeal of foods, contrasts with most food groups and has been used as a plate colour for many decades (Timlin and Rysenbry, 2010).

The essential point is to focus attention on the most important part of the meal – the food. Some of the best plate-design features include an outer ring of colour around the edge of the plate (Timlin and Rysenbry, 2010), helping to distinguish the edge of the plate from the table and focusing the attention on that important stuff in the middle of the plate; one example is a dark navy blue plate with a white outer rim.

Finally when considering colour contrast at the table setting it may not be necessary to change the colour of the plate as a tablecloth may provide the necessary contrast. For example a dark blue tablecloth and white plate with silver cutlery provides high contrast, making identifying/seeing the plate and cutlery much easier. An additional benefit of changing the tablecloth is that it can make the table look more attractive and homelike.

Tableware, colour contrast and lighting

An additional factor when providing contrast and aiding visual cueing at the mealtime is the importance of adjusting the lighting in the environment. General lighting requirements at the mealtime are discussed in Chapter 10 whereas the evidence for lighting improving eating abilities and food intake is discussed now.

Multicomponent intervention approaches using the addition of light and high contrast tableware led to improved nutritional intake, more engagement, improved eating abilities and less agitated behaviour in care home residents with dementia (Brush, Meehan and Calkins, 2002). Here the researchers chose to use a navy blue tray liner under the white plates and also a dark green tablecloth, although the tablecloth was mainly to cover peeling and unattractive tables. Of note, it might be better to avoid putting blue and green together, as apart from them being garish, blue colours can appear more like green to an eye with visual clarity problems (Jakob and Collier, 2013).

In a reported case study from a dementia care home, yellow plates on maroon placemats and enhanced lighting led to a slight decrease in food consumption, perhaps due to a lack of contrast between the yellow plate and the food (Brush, Fleder and Calkins, 2012). Owing to this the intervention was changed to red plates on a white placemat, again with enhanced lighting, with 26 individuals increasing food intake, 14 decreasing intake and 23 maintaining intake. This real-life case study showed that interventions do not work the same for everyone; therefore changing all your plates to one particular colour can be detrimental. Many organisations have adopted coloured plates for all people with dementia in an attempt to improve their nutrition.

This case study however stresses the importance of reviewing outcomes and also tailoring interventions to the person rather than adopting a blanket approach to cover care for everyone.

The most important thing at the dinner table is the food; please let's not forget this. Modify the tableware so that all attention is drawn to the food, making it easy to distinguish. This will take different forms of interventions for different people and may require multiple modifications. The box below provides a summary of practical approaches for enhancing tableware using colour contrast. Also, although adapting the colour contrast of drinking beverages has not been studied the same contrast methods can be applied here.

Tips on using colour contrast tableware

Provide contrast between the plate and table
Coloured plates and tablecloths can be used, for example a blue plate on a white tablecloth (or white plate on a blue tablecloth or dark table finish). Different-coloured placemats can provide a similar effect.

Provide a high colour contrast between the plate and the food
For example the edge of a plate can have a different contrast to the centre, such as a dark blue plate with a white rim or coloured plates. Alternatively the food can be of high contrast to the colour of the plate.

Do not change the tableware
Instead present a variety of coloured foods in attractive ways.

Use a combination of all three approaches
Another addition is suitable lighting at a mealtime, which has been shown to enhance the colour contrast provided by the tableware.

Tableware to support eating abilities

Whereas modifying tableware to provide contrast can help with visual cueing to eat, tableware can also be used to make the process of eating less complex. Cleverly designed tableware can provide the assistance someone requires to continue to feed themselves rather than relying on the assistance from a carer to be fed. For example a 'Reduced ability to get food onto cutlery (spoon, fork or knife)' (see the list of common self-feeding abilities at the beginning of this chapter) means someone may be observed repeatedly using the wrong end of the cutlery to try to pick up some food. This may lead to them being fed by a carer as they are not eating their food. However, adaptive cutlery can be provided like a 'spork' (spoon head on one end and fork head on the other end) which will allow the person to continue self-feeding and preserve this eating ability. Further examples of supportive tableware include suction plates or non-slip mats which prevent the plate from sliding on the table. These mats are often coloured and in addition to preventing the plate moving may provide a colour contrast, as discussed above; they were used to good effect in one study (Brush et al., 2012). The use of this equipment means a carer is not required to support the plate while the person eats, allowing them to focus on others who may actually need assistance. Other examples include adaptive cutlery to enable easier meat cutting ('Reduced ability to cut meat (or other foods)'), cutlery with large handles or additional grip, or 'scoop plates' or plate guards making it easier to get food onto the cutlery ('Reduced ability to get food onto cutlery (spoon, fork or knife)'). In the simplest terms just providing a spoon and scoop plate and reducing the complex options available at a meal may provide the right conditions for someone to continue eating without additional assistance. Unfortunately evidence for the effectiveness of these practical interventions is lacking despite their widespread use in care settings.

Tableware to support drinking abilities

The importance of finding ingenious ways to promote hydration in people with dementia cannot be overemphasised. The consequences of dehydration can contribute to increased symptoms of dementia and increase the risk of other complications such as falls, urinary tract infections and constipation (Reed et al., 2005), all of which decrease the quality of life for the person and make providing care even more complex. There is very little research evidence on what specific interventions carers can put in place to ensure adequate fluid intake in people with dementia who have reduced drinking abilities (Ullrich and McCutcheon, 2008). Modifying drinking equipment can be one specific intervention to try.

When thinking about adapted drinking containers used in dementia care, visions of cups that look like baby beakers inevitably spring to mind. Clearly design has a long way to go in dementia care to make eating and drinking utensils look more sophisticated and less childlike. Cleverly designed tableware products are available as described in *Design for Dementia: Improving Dining and Bedroom Environments in Care Homes* (Timlin and Rysenbry, 2010, pp.35–9). Despite the lack of sophisticated design many adapted tableware products for drinking can be useful in supporting abilities. If you observe someone with a 'Reduced ability using cups or glasses' or who 'Spills drinks when drinking' there is a range of supportive tableware available to help. Preferably before reaching for the enlarged plastic baby cup see if they can continue to drink themselves when using a cup with extra grip, or a cup with a large handle or two handles which are still made out of crockery rather than plastic.

Whereas there has been some research looking at the effect on food intake of modifying tableware through contrast and lighting there is nothing on repeating these techniques for improving fluid intake. This does not mean they are ineffective or should be discounted but be aware that monitoring of their effectiveness as with all interventions is imperative.

Swallowing difficulties and modifying drinking equipment

Swallowing difficulties are discussed in detail in Chapter 8 but there are a few important considerations related to swallowing difficulties and using modified drinking equipment. If someone has a swallowing difficulty then the position of the head when drinking becomes important to minimise the risks of aspiration or choking. Keeping the chin level is also recommended. For example most spouted beakers require the person to tip their head back significantly and should be avoided. A wide or shallow cup which prevents the need to tip the head back would be more suitable (Kellett, 2012).

In general, straws can be useful in enabling someone to maintain fluid intake who finds using drinking equipment troublesome. With a swallowing difficulty straws can also help keep the chin level when drinking. However, there are some important considerations and it is necessary to be aware of any signs of difficulty (Kellett, 2012):

- Using a straw with a delayed or weak swallow could increase the risk of aspiration of liquid into the lungs.

- A straw should never be used in a reclined position if a better posture is possible.

- Not everybody is able to suck effectively through a straw although valved straws can help a person with a weak suck.

A speech and language therapist will help determine the appropriate use of straws in someone with dementia and a swallowing difficulty.

Summary of modifying tableware

Modified tableware is easily accessible to all carers and can be tailored to the person's needs if the correct assessment of their mealtime abilities is made. Individual assessment will also prevent interventions being put in place that may hinder rather than support abilities. This is an important point as the limited research indicates that these types of interventions may not work in the majority of people with dementia. For example, changing the colour of the plate with little thought about the actual colour contrast between plate and food will likely lead to less food being eaten by some. Using enhanced lighting with a change in colour contrast may provide more benefit than just changing the contrast. Older people can require three times as much light as younger people but are more sensitive to glare. It is important to remember that achieving a well-lit dining area and avoiding areas of dim lighting or glare can potentially enhance the effectiveness of using colour contrast tableware. Enabling the person with dementia to see as clearly as possible through careful use of colour and position of objects to accommodate visual problems can also improve their quality of life (Armstrong, 2009).

When using adaptive eating and drinking equipment it may take time for some people to become used to this; therefore monitoring the effects of any adaptations is important. The design of eating and drinking equipment modified for use by people with dementia needs to improve to reduce its plastic and childlike appearance. There is however more modified tableware available that looks just like 'normal' tableware.

Finally, when considering modified tableware we must ensure that the person is positioned correctly to actually see and be able to eat the food in front of them. This is not strictly related to dementia but rather more general advice.

Positioning

Adaptive eating and drinking equipment can be a simple and effective intervention but it is also important that the person is correctly positioned at mealtimes. Improving their position may eliminate the need for modified tableware. Observing those who have positioning problems should indicate the need for further assessment. If someone has chronic difficulties getting in the correct position then an occupational therapist can provide an assessment and advice on correct positioning and modified furniture if appropriate, along with specific adaptive tableware.

Correct positioning is particularly important if someone has a swallowing difficulty as poor positioning can increase the chances of an adverse event occurring such as aspiration or choking. Positioning for those with swallowing difficulties is discussed briefly in Chapter 8. A speech and language therapist should always be consulted on the best position at the mealtime for each individual to help ensure their safe and effective swallowing.

The carer's position in relation to the person they are assisting is also important (Ullrich and McCutcheon, 2008). Sitting in the prominent position in front of them face to face at a 90-degree angle so they are in the line of sight is best but can be practically difficult to achieve. Making sure you as a carer are comfortable as well as the person you are helping is just as important as sitting on a level with them so that your presence is not intimidating (Kellett, 2012).

Adapting Meals – finger foods

To support people with dementia there are many adaptations to food that can be trialled. In this section on self-feeding abilities the use of finger foods is typically the predominant intervention.

Finger foods are those that can be eaten without cutlery and can form the basis of all food consumed if required and appropriate. There is plenty of literature that provides information on the use of finger foods in dementia; see other practical documents (Crawley and Hocking, 2011) and books (Morgan-Jones et al., 2016) which provide useful information. Despite the use of finger foods being advocated for many years there is often still a lack of choice on menus in care homes or hospital. When finger foods are used they can be rather dull with little imagination put into their creation, with a reliance on things such as sausage rolls. This is where the work now needs to take place to ensure there is not only a range of suitable finger foods but also finger foods with a texture-modified form for those who have swallowing difficulties and have reduced abilities to eat using traditional cutlery. Certainly limited research on the use of finger foods in people with dementia has shown that their attractiveness and the choice available both positively affect consumption (Pouyet et al., 2014). Finger foods have also been shown to prevent further weight loss in people with dementia (Alibhai, Greenwood and Payette, 2005). Please make sure the person has the opportunity to wash their hands if finger foods are being offered, or at least use a disinfectant hand gel.

Further interventions and referrals

Increasing socialisation at mealtimes by eating meals with someone or modifying the serving style to increase interaction are further possible interventions for improving self-feeding abilities and food intake. These interventions are included in Chapter 5 but are discussed in detail in Chapter 6.

If a range of interventions have been tried and monitored and someone's abilities have not been maintained then further assistance such as physical feeding may be required. A referral to an occupational therapist for further advice on enhancing eating abilities may also be indicated. If the reduction in eating abilities impacts too on the person's food intake or causes weight loss and puts them at risk of malnutrition a referral to a dietitian is warranted.

Promoting dignity

All the interventions discussed in this section can have a direct impact on not only enhancing independence at mealtimes but also helping to promote mealtime dignity for the person with dementia.

This is particularly important when we think of providing feeding assistance. It has been noted that a common response by carers to reduced mealtime abilities is to provide increased feeding assistance. This may actually increase the dependence on receiving assistance and ideally people with dementia should only be provided with a level of assistance actually required to consume their food in a safe and dignified manner (Lin et al., 2010).

Specifically related to dignity and often used with people with later stage dementia is protective clothing. The use of protective clothing, aprons or bibs is to prevent someone from soiling their clothes as food spillage is common. Some of these items however can be seen to be offensive to the person concerned and may contribute to increased meal behaviours such as refusal to eat. Large napkins can be used instead and there are also some very attractive scarf bibs or cravats that can help preserve someone's dignity if they require something to prevent food spilling on themselves. If the person you care for has, or was known for having, a sense of humour you can even get personalised adult bibs stating 'Dinners On Me!' A large shirt or something similar can also be used rather than a bib and may help preserve self-esteem. Assessing someone for the required support at mealtime – whether it is with their position, cueing or modified tableware – will help reduce food spillage and maintain dignity (National Food Service Management Institute, 2005a).

Summary

There are many interventions that can be put in place to support eating and drinking abilities that can lead to enhanced independence, dignity and quality of life. It is clear however that all interventions will require additional caring time if they are to be effective. Research authors have noted how lack of time and other caring responsibilities may be confounding factors for the success of mealtime interventions (Ullrich and McCutcheon, 2008). Indeed this barrier to improved mealtime care can be associated with the type of care training provided to carers. The role of mealtime care training is traditionally focused on facilitating feeding along with the safety and positioning techniques associated with feeding. Mealtimes can therefore become focused on the task of feeding rather than providing support for eating and drinking abilities through the process described in this and the next chapter. Providing additional support to people with dementia to help them maintain independence rather than foster dependence involves many caring skills that may have been neglected in training.

To support people living with later-stage dementia to maintain independence and continue to feed themselves for as long as possible there is a process of assessment and interventions that can be put in place. Assessment should start at the mealtime, observing and learning what the specific needs of the person are. Interventions should start with simple cueing techniques and move on to more advanced cueing techniques. Progression of interventions towards modifying tableware or the mealtime setting to enhance the current level of eating ability, and making adaptations to the texture of food and alterations in the environment, can continue to preserve some independence. As more assistance becomes necessary, using hand feeding techniques at the level required assists the person to continue self-feeding before eventually full feeding assistance may be required. Before this time a referral to an occupational therapist may be indicated for additional support and guidance. Importantly, learning how to put all these processes in place will help guide carers to focus on the person with dementia and what their needs are, which will always help in providing the most appropriate person-centred care.

The next chapter (the first of four practical chapters: 5, 7, 9 and 11) will provide simple, practical and cost-effective suggestions based on the available evidence described in this chapter.

5

Practical Interventions Section 1

ENHANCING INDEPENDENCE AND DIGNITY AT MEALTIMES

Assessment and interventions: independence and dignity at mealtimes

To respond to the needs of someone with dementia at a mealtime you first need to assess their needs. Without an in-depth knowledge of dementia and dementia care it can be very hard for carers to identify these needs, which are often observed as reduced eating and drinking abilities. In addition, having the knowledge to then provide a range of interventions to support those needs is clearly even harder. The practical intervention chapters (5, 7, 9 and 11) will provide a systematic way first to assess and second to intervene to support the specific identified needs.

Assessment

Even though the reduction in abilities related to independence and dignity at mealtimes is common it is not commonly assessed, and so is not recognised by carers and can go unsupported. This leads to a further reduction in the ability to self-feed and ultimately the person with dementia ends up being fed by a carer rather than feeding themselves. Assessment therefore is the first crucial step in supporting the abilities needed to eat and drink. The abilities listed in Table 5.1

are found in several of the mealtime assessment tools described in Chapter 3. These tools are not widely or freely available and different assessment tools would be needed to be used to cover the range of eating and drinking abilities observed. For a simple and practical assessment of these abilities and other mealtime abilities the use of the Dementia Mealtime Assessment Tool (the DMAT) is recommended.

Section 1 of the DMAT (DMAT, 2017) is reproduced in Table 5.1 and can be used to assess self-feeding eating and drinking abilities. This chapter uses section 1 of four from the DMAT while the full version of the DMAT is included in Chapter 3 and is available freely online (DMAT, 2017). If the correct assessment of self-feeding abilities is made at this time then these abilities can be preserved or enhanced.

Table 5.1: The DMAT section 1: Assessment of self-feeding abilities

	Please tick observed abilities		
Mealtime observations: Abilities to self-feed	Not seen	Seen once	Seen repeatedly
1. Reduced ability to use cutlery (spoon, fork or knife)			
2. Reduced ability to get food onto cutlery (spoon, fork or knife)			
3. Reduced ability to cut meat (or other foods)			
4. Reduced ability in identifying food from plate			
5. Plate slides or is moved around the table			
6. Reduced ability using cups or glasses			
7. Reduced ability seeing or identifying cups or glasses			
8. Spills drinks when drinking			
9. Stares at food without eating			
10. Falls asleep or is asleep during mealtime			

The carer should use recommendations in Chapter 3 and the guidance below when using the DMAT to assess current self-feeding abilities by observing the person with dementia at a mealtime and simply ticking the appropriate boxes of observed abilities. Once the assessment has been made then a carer can choose the most appropriate interventions to support the reduced abilities from the range listed in this chapter.

Interventions

The interventions used to enhance self-feeding abilities should start with the simplest, non-invasive and least assistance and then proceed on to more complex interventions requiring increased assistance and eventually ending with complete assistance (Coyne and Hoskins, 1997). Although these types of interventions will require more time initially to implement, their systematic use can encourage self-feeding, which is the key to independence and dignity at mealtimes.

Remember that the type of intervention or level of support provided to someone can change from day to day (Ullrich and McCutcheon, 2008). The amount of assistance required may be less or more and carers will need to be aware of these sometimes subtle changes so they support the person in the most appropriate way. For example this may mean adapting their usual approach and concentrating on improving abilities more reduced on that particular day.

Read the guidance below before attempting any of the interventions provided in the following interventions list.

Guidance for interventions

- All the interventions are aimed at simplifying the process of eating.

- All interventions are based on available evidence and best-practice guidelines discussed throughout the book, sometimes with a practical adaptation.

- All the interventions can and should form part of common care practices.

- Interventions will overlap in their use in different eating and drinking abilities.

- Each intervention starts with a 'category' label indicating the main type of intervention; for example the intervention is based on 'cueing' techniques or 'modifying tableware'.

- It may be more effective to only implement one or two interventions at a time.

- Allow four weeks for evaluation of the effectiveness of the chosen intervention and use the DMAT again four weeks later to reassess any changes in eating abilities.

- Record and monitor the intervention used and outcomes achieved, for example in a care plan.

- IMPORTANT NOTICE: Some reduced abilities can indicate further assessment may be required or that the patient may be at increased risk at mealtimes. If this is the case for the list of interventions available to enhance this reduced ability an 'IMPORTANT NOTICE' will be highlighted at the start of the intervention list. It is important both to read and understand what this means in relation to the person who is being cared for, and to act appropriately to prevent any harm to the person.

- CARE HOME SPECIFIC: The vast majority of suggested interventions can be applied to different settings, for example home care, care home, acute care, independent living and so on. However, the majority of research has been conducted in care home or long-term care settings, and some interventions will only be applicable to these settings and will be labelled 'CARE HOME SPECIFIC'.

- REFERRAL: As labelled, if several interventions have been attempted but the mealtime ability has not been enhanced, then this would indicate a referral to the appropriate healthcare professional.

Suggested interventions for supporting eating and drinking abilities to enhance independence and dignity at mealtimes

1. Reduced ability to use cutlery (spoon, fork or knife)

- Provide cueing:
  - Offer verbal cues and verbal prompting, for example 'Pick up your fork', to help the person initiate use of cutlery. Also offer encouragement.

- Manually show correct use of cutlery by 'modelling' the task a few times; for example use your fork to pretend to eat, so the person can copy your movements. Also offer encouragement.

- Place food or utensils in the person's hand and trial using hand-over-hand or hand-under-hand technique to initiate and guide self-feeding. Also offer encouragement.

- Try reminiscence therapy to engage the person in conversation to see if this enhances the eating ability.

- Trial eating meals with the person so that they can follow your lead and initiate self-feeding. Also offer encouragement.

- Trial using hand-over-hand or preferably hand-under-hand technique to intitiate and guide self-feeding. Also offer encouragement.

- Modify table setting:

  - Limit the number of utensils. Simplify the cutlery by only having a spoon available and ensure all food can be eaten using a spoon.

- Modify tableware:

  - Trial using adapted cutlery, for example large-handled cutlery with extra grip. Also offer encouragement.

  - Trial using adapted cutlery, for example 'all in one' spoon and fork on the same utensil. Also offer encouragement.

  - Trial using a scoop plate and spoon for continued self-feeding rather than a plate and cutlery. Also offer encouragement.

- Increase socialisation:

  - Try eating your meal with the person. Eating with company can enhance mealtime abilities owing to social interaction and taking cues to eat from others. In addition you can help keep their focus on the meal and provide appropriate assistance if required to help maintain food intake.

- Adapting the service style of food may improve the eating ability, for example sharing meals at the table or providing the opportunity to serve their own food. This can also improve portion size and food choice.

- Adapt food:

    - Trial finger foods which will help take the pressure off using cutlery to eat.

- Full assistance:

    - If all suggestions fail then the person may require assistance with feeding. Therefore trial full feeding assistance for two days and record and monitor food and fluid intake at mealtimes.

- CARE HOME SPECIFIC: Increase socialisation:

    - Consider seating arrangements. Sit the person with a friend or someone they have an affinity with to enhance social interaction which may improve abilities. Or if already doing this sit them with someone who has maintained eating abilities, as this may help the person continue to feed themselves by taking cues from others.

- REFERRAL: Consult with an occupational therapist for further assessment of specific eating needs.

2. Reduced ability to get food onto cutlery (spoon, fork or knife)

- Modify table setting:

    - Limit the number of utensils. Simplify the cutlery by only having a spoon available and ensure all food can be eaten using a spoon.

- Modify tableware:

    - A deeper spoon may help the food stay on the cutlery better than a flatter spoon.

- Trial using adapted cutlery, for example large-handled cutlery with extra grip. Also offer encouragement.

- Trial using adapted cutlery, for example an 'all in one' spoon and fork on the same utensil. Also offer encouragement.

- Trial a plate guard or lipped plate (also called a scoop plate) to make it easier to scoop up food. Also offer encouragement.

- Provide cueing:

  - Trial using hand-over-hand or preferably hand-under-hand technique to initiate and guide self-feeding. Also offer encouragement.

- Adapt food:

  - Trial finger foods which will help take the pressure off using cutlery to eat.

- CARE HOME SPECIFIC: Increase socialisation:

  - Consider seating arrangements. Sit the person with a friend or someone they have an affinity with to enhance social interaction which may improve abilities. Or if already doing this sit them with someone who has maintained eating abilities, as this may help the person continue to feed themselves by taking cues from others.

- REFERRAL: Consult with an occupational therapist for further assessment of specific eating needs

3. Reduced ability to cut meat (or other foods)

- Modify tableware:

  - Trial adapted cutlery such as knives that use a rocking rather than sawing motion (this could particularly help those with a reduced grip strength). Also offer encouragement.

- Adapt food:

  - Provide meals with cut meats (or other pre-cut foods if needed).

- Trial softer meats and foods to see if this makes the task easier.

- Trial finger foods which will help take the pressure off using cutlery to eat.

• REFERRAL: Consult with an occupational therapist for further assessment of specific eating needs.

4. Reduced ability in identifying food from plate

• Provide cueing:

- Check glasses are worn if normally used to assist vision.

- Offer verbal cues and verbal prompting; for example tell the person what they are eating and where it is on the plate. Also offer encouragement.

- Manually show and correct the person to help them identify the food. Also offer encouragement.

• Modify table setting:

- Assist vision by making sure objects (salt and pepper pots, glasses, placemats, etc.) are not too close together or on top of each other, as they may appear blended together.

- Clear non-food clutter from table.

• Modify tableware:

- Ensure a high colour contrast between the plate and the food thereby making it easier to visualise.

- Trial using plates with a simple plain design, for example a white plate with a blue-rimmed edge. This can help define the differences between the table, plate and food.

- Trial a colour contrast between the table or placemat and the plate of food; for example a white plate on a white tablecloth may make identifying the food harder. Note: tablecloths make dining more attractive and may provide the colour contrast required rather than changing the plate colour.

- Adjust environment:

  - Adjust the lighting to assist vision. People living with dementia tend to need increased light compared to normal. Try to achieve high levels of illumination in mealtime areas while still maintaining a homely feel.

  - Reduce glare from natural or electric lights to assist vision. If seated near a window the outside light may cause glare (especially if reflected from shiny surfaces) making it harder to see the meal; therefore try moving the meal place or reduce surfaces that cause glare, for example by using a tablecloth on a shiny table.

- REFERRAL: Consult with an occupational therapist for further assessment of specific eating needs.

5. Plate slides or is moved around the table

- Modify tableware:

  - Trial the use of a non-slip placemat or tray.

  - Trial the use of a suction plate.

  - Trial a plate guard or lipped plate (also called a scoop plate) to make it easier to scoop up food.

- Provide cueing:

  - Assist at mealtimes by supporting the plate and allowing the person to continue feeding themselves.

- REFERRAL: Consult with an occupational therapist for further assessment of specific eating needs.

6. Reduced ability using cups or glasses

- IMPORTANT NOTICE: If the person has dysphagia (swallowing difficulty) then an incorrect head position at mealtimes is a high-risk factor for a negative health consequence (asphyxiation and/or choking episode, aspiration incidents, dehydration and poor nutritional status). Be extra vigilant when using spouted beakers or straws.

- Provide cueing:

  - Offer verbal cues and verbal prompting to explain use of cups or glasses. Also offer encouragement.

  - Manually show use of cup or glass so the person can copy your movements. Also offer encouragement.

  - Try reminiscence therapy to engage the person in conversation to see if this enhances their drinking ability.

  - Trial using hand-over-hand or preferably hand-under-hand technique to initiate and guide self-feeding. Also offer encouragement.

- Modify tableware:

  - Trial using drinking equipment with additional grip. Also offer encouragement.

  - Lighter plastic cups may be easier to use. Also offer encouragement.

  - Trial using drinking equipment with a large handle or two handles for easier use. Also offer encouragement.

  - Trial the use of a straw, for example a uniflow straw, if picking up the drinking equipment is too hard. If the person has a swallowing difficulty check if a straw should be used.

  - Trial using a non-spill mug with lid and spout if acceptable. Also offer encouragement.

- Adapt drinks:

  - Some drinks can be offered as frozen lollies on sticks or as a sorbet in cones if drinking becomes stressful. Also offer encouragement.

- Adapt food:

  - Some foods have a naturally high water content, for example soup, jelly, custard, sauces, watermelon or similar fruits and yoghurt. Therefore offer more of these types of foods if drinking enough fluid is problematic, and provide encouragement.

- Increase socialisation:
  - Try offering drinks in a social setting to see if this improves ability. Social interaction can increase intake and enhance abilities through copying others.

  - Try eating your meal with the person. Eating with company can enhance mealtime abilities owing to social interaction and taking cues to eat from others. In addition you can help keep their focus on the meal and provide appropriate assistance if required to help maintain food intake.

- Full assistance:
  - Try providing water by using a spoon. This may result in a slow but sustained intake of fluid.

- CARE HOME SPECIFIC: Increase socialisation:
  - Consider seating arrangements. Sit the person with a friend or someone they have an affinity with to enhance social interaction, which may improve abilities. Or if already doing this sit them with someone who has maintained eating abilities as this may help the person continue to feed themselves by taking cues from others.

- REFERRAL: Consult with an occupational therapist for further assessment of specific eating needs.

7. Reduced ability seeing or identifying cups or glasses

- IMPORTANT NOTICE: If the person has dysphagia (swallowing difficulty) then an incorrect head position at mealtimes is a high-risk factor for a negative health consequence (asphyxiation and/or choking episode, aspiration incidents, dehydration and poor nutritional status). Be extra vigilant when using spouted beakers or straws.

- Modify table setting:

  - Assist vision by ensuring cups or glasses are within the person's field of vision (their visionary field may be very narrow and focused to what is directly in front of them).

- Provide cueing:

  - Offer verbal cues and verbal prompting to help the person identify the cups or glasses. Also offer encouragement.

  - Manually show the cup or glass so the person is aware of its location. Also offer encouragement.

  - Put the cup/glass into the person's hand to prompt them to drink, rather than leaving it on the table. Also offer encouragement.

- Adapt drinks:

  - Trial coloured liquids in a glass, for example squash, as this may be more noticeable than water.

- Modify tableware:

  - Trial using coloured cups and glasses, ensuring they have a colour contrast to the table or tablecloth.

- Adjust environment:

  - Adjust the lighting to assist vision. People living with dementia tend to need increased light compared to normal. Try to achieve high levels of illumination in mealtime areas while still maintaining a homely feel.

  - Reduce glare from natural or electric lights to assist vision. If seated near a window the outside light may cause glare (especially if reflected from shiny surfaces) making it harder to see the meal; therefore try moving the meal place or reduce surfaces that cause glare, for example by using a tablecloth on a shiny table.

- REFERRAL: Consult with an occupational therapist for further assessment of specific eating needs.

8. Spills drinks when drinking

- IMPORTANT NOTICE: If the person has dysphagia (swallowing difficulty) then an incorrect head position at mealtimes is a high-risk factor for a negative health consequence (asphyxiation and/or choking episode, aspiration incidents, dehydration and poor nutritional status). Be extra vigilant when using spouted beakers or straws.

- Modify tableware:
  - Offer small amounts of fluid at a time in a stable cup with a handle the person can easily grip. Also offer encouragement.
  - Trial using drinking equipment with additional grip. Also offer encouragement.
  - Lighter plastic cups may be easier to use. Also offer encouragement.
  - Trial using drinking equipment with a large handle or two handles for easier use. Also offer encouragement.
  - Trial the use of a straw, for example a uniflow straw, if picking up the drinking equipment is too hard. If the person has a swallowing difficulty check if a straw should be used.
  - Trial using a non-spill mug with lid and spout if acceptable. Also offer encouragement.

- Provide cueing:
  - Trial using hand-over-hand or preferably hand-under-hand technique to initiate and guide self-feeding. Also offer encouragement.

- Adapt drinks:
  - Some drinks can be offered as frozen lollies on sticks or as a sorbet in cones if drinking becomes stressful. Also offer encouragement.

- Adapt food:
  - Some foods have a naturally high water content, for example soup, jelly, custard, sauces, watermelon or similar

fruits and yoghurt. Therefore offer more of these types of foods if drinking enough fluid is problematic, and provide encouragement.

- REFERRAL: Consult with an occupational therapist for further assessment of specific eating needs.

9. Stares at food without eating

- Provide cueing:
  - Verbally reassure and remind the person where they are, what time it is and what they are doing.
  - Check hearing aids or glasses are worn if normally used.
  - Offer verbal cues and prompting to help the person initiate eating, for example 'How is your food?' Also offer encouragement.
  - Try reminiscence therapy to engage the person in conversation to see if this triggers them to start eating.
  - Try manual cues, for example placing food or utensils into the person's hands. Also offer encouragement.
  - Try modelling eating so the person can copy your movements. Also offer encouragement.
  - Try a more expressive act such as gently touching the forearm or gently rubbing the top of the person's hand to get their attention and then focus them on the meal.
  - Trial using hand-over-hand or preferably hand-under-hand technique to initiate and guide self-feeding. Also offer encouragement.
- Modify table setting:
  - Simplify the meal process by placing only one plate and one utensil on the table, directly in front of the person. When they are finished with the first dish, replace it with another. Also offer encouragement.

- Modify tableware:

  - Ensure a high colour contrast between the plate and the food thereby making it easier to visualise.

  - Trial using plates with a simple plain design, for example a white plate with a blue rimmed edge. This can help define the differences between the table, plate and food.

  - Trial a colour contrast between the table or placemat and the plate; for example a white plate on a white tablecloth may make identifying the food harder. *Note:* tablecloths make dining more attractive and may provide the colour contrast required rather than changing the plate colour.

- Adjust environment:

  - Adjust the lighting to assist vision. People living with dementia tend to need increased light compared to normal. Try to achieve high levels of illumination in mealtime areas while still maintaining a homely feel.

  - Reduce glare from natural or electric lights to assist vision. If seated near a window the outside light may cause glare (especially if reflected from shiny surfaces) making it harder to see the meal; therefore try moving the meal place or reduce surfaces that cause glare, for example by using a tablecloth on a shiny table.

- Increase socialisation:

  - Try eating your meal with the person. Eating with company can enhance mealtime abilities owing to social interaction and taking cues to eat from others. In addition you can help keep their focus on the meal and provide appropriate assistance if required to help maintain food intake.

  - Adapting the service style of food may improve eating ability, for example sharing meals at the table or providing the opportunity to serve their own food. This can also improve portion size and food choice.

- CARE HOME SPECIFIC: Consider seating arrangements. Sit the person with a friend or someone they have an affinity with to enhance social interaction, which may improve abilities. Or if already doing this sit them with someone who has maintained eating abilities as this may help the person continue to feed themselves by taking cues from others.

- REFERRAL: If the person continues not to eat, provide feeding assistance and consult with a dietitian for nutritional assessment.

10. Falls asleep or is asleep during mealtime

- IMPORTANT NOTICE: If the person has dysphagia (swallowing difficulty) then reduced alertness and cooperation at meal-times is a high-risk factor for a negative health consequence (asphyxiation and/or choking episode, aspiration incidents, dehydration and poor nutritional status). Do not attempt to force-feed the person.

- Provide cueing:

  - Ensure the person is prepared and aware that it is nearly mealtime. Allow time for them to become alert and awake.

  - Gently pat the person's face with a cool damp cloth to increase their alertness.

  - Try manual cues and verbal prompting to help the person initiate eating again. Also offer encouragement.

  - Try a more expressive act such as gently touching the forearm or gently rubbing the top of the person's hand to get their attention and then focus them on the meal.

- Adjust environment:

  - Adjust the lighting to assist vision. People living with dementia tend to need increased light compared to normal. Try to achieve high levels of illumination in mealtime areas while still maintaining a homely feel.

- IMPORTANT NOTICE: Do not attempt to force-feed someone. Following several attempts to prompt them to eat, if they are still asleep or drowsy then stop the meal to prevent distressing them.

- CARE HOME SPECIFIC: Increase socialisation:
  - Consider seating arrangements. Sit the person with a friend or someone they have an affinity with to enhance social interaction, which may improve abilities. Or if already doing this sit them with someone who has maintained eating abilities as this may help the person continue to feed themselves by taking cues from others.

- REFERRAL: Consider a medication review if the person is often asleep during the day. Consult with a doctor.

6

Preferences and Choice at Mealtimes

THE SENSORY EXPERIENCE

Introduction

People with dementia living in nursing homes have voiced their concerns and frustrations regarding both their individual needs and preferences for dietary care not being met, and the barriers they perceive to receiving dietary care to meet these needs and preferences. They have also described a loss of control and choice available, especially for those with reduced mealtime abilities and swallowing difficulties (Milte *et al.*, 2017). The authors of this research highlighted that to really provide person-centred care and support quality of life then more consideration must be given to individualised dietary care. This book is providing one of many ways to achieve this through evidence-based assessment and interventions, with the focus of this chapter and the following practical interventions chapter being preferences and choice at mealtimes.

Preferences with regards to how food and fluid are consumed change as dementia advances to later stages. The list below shows some commonly observed preferences with eating and drinking as dementia progresses, along with some meal behaviours and changes in mealtime abilities related to meal preferences and choice. This list is taken from section 2 of the Dementia Mealtime Assessment Tool (DMAT).

Common preferences with eating and drinking that can affect food and fluid intake

- Prefers sweet food or eats desserts/sweets first

- Only eats certain foods

- Eats (or drinks) too fast

- Mixes food together

- Does not eat lunch but eats breakfast and some dinner

- Eats very small amounts of food (or drink)

- Slow eating or prolonged mealtimes

Adapted from Durnbaugh et al. (1996); Watson (1996); Crawley and Hocking (2011)

Two of the most common changes determining a person's preferences include a preference for sweeter foods, as the ability to taste food changes, and consuming smaller portion sizes of meals because of reduced satiety levels. These mean that when catering for older people with dementia there are many additional elements to consider; it is important not only to provide a variety of choice but also to provide tasty and nutritious meals. Another catering challenge is that these meals may need to be in the form of finger foods, have soft or purée options and have stronger flavours.

The interventions in this section will discuss some clever methods of using tableware, supplying food fortification, changing meal patterns, providing food little and often, and adapting taste and smell to ensure optimum nutritional intake.

The evidence for augmenting preferences with eating and drinking

Before reviewing the evidence on specific interventions to support preferences with food intake it is important to remember that there is only a small amount of evidence available despite widespread use of many interventions in care settings. This lack of research is a constant hindrance to those trying to provide better nutritional care for people living with dementia. However, as systematic reviews of this evidence have indicated, carers still need to provide care at mealtimes and find ways to meet the nutritional requirements of people living with dementia despite the lack of effectiveness of the interventions currently used (Abdelhamid *et al.*, 2016).

Practical observations, clinical experience and research evidence all point to the fact that you can provide plenty of food and even prescribe oral nutrition supplements (that provide far in excess of the energy requirements for someone with dementia) yet this does not result in increased intake of those calories (Leslie *et al.*, 2013). This is especially true in those with a low body mass index (BMI) at whom these nutrition interventions are targeted (Young, Binns and Greenwood, 2001).

Providing energy-dense and nutritious food is obviously important but if the food is not eaten it has no nutritional value. There are already good sources of information explaining ways to increase calories and nutrients in food to provide better nutritional value (Crawley and Hocking, 2011). Additionally if there is access to a dietitian then this general nutritional fortification advice can be tailored to the individual.

After making these nutritional changes what if the person with dementia is still not eating? This chapter focuses on the practical issues of supporting people with dementia to eat the food rather than the nutrient profile of the food you are providing. It is extremely important that the types of food and food service are optimised to suit the preferences of people living with dementia, especially for those at risk of malnutrition.

Cueing and choice
Cueing
As discussed in detail in Chapter 4, using cueing techniques is a useful starting point when supporting people with dementia at mealtimes. The same principles discussed when using verbal, manual and other forms of prompting and encouragement in Chapter 5 should be applied to encouraging consumption of food and fluid in line with personal preferences. The cueing intervention examples outlined in Chapter 7 are all simple and practical suggestions and are not related to any specific research studies.

Choice

Unfortunately offering choice can be overlooked as a method of cueing a person living with dementia. Providing choice may simply be enough to improve their intake. In a study looking at interactions at mealtime between carers and care home residents with dementia this autonomy of offering choice was the least-observed interaction, falling behind cueing, encouragement and coaxing (Ullrich and McCutcheon, 2008). Often those with more cognitive ability were the ones offered a choice when clearly, just because your dementia has progressed more than someone else's, it does not mean you would not like a choice of food or drink. When considering preferences with food and drink the importance of choice cannot be emphasised enough. Those in the early stages of dementia have indicated they wished to have choice of when and what they ate and not be part of a set daily routine, along with having opportunities for social interaction at mealtimes (Timlin and Rysenbry, 2010).

In a busy mealtime environment it can be almost impossible to work out someone's preferences and help identify appropriate choices. Over time if the same carer is providing the mealtime care then likes and dislikes may be discovered; however, during this lengthy process nutritional intake may suffer. Having knowledge of the person's past preferences may help although as dementia advances and preferences change this may not be as useful. There are nonetheless some very practical ways to help identify choices and preferences for food and drink.

PICTURE MENUS

Using picture menus, that is, pictures of the food served at mealtimes, can be a useful way of offering choices, as a picture will be easier to understand and identify than verbal descriptions. Having said this some people with poorer vision may find it easier to see pictures of single food items rather than an image of a finished meal. Using picture menus as a way of offering choice is more suitable for those with mild dementia but it is also important that the pictures reflect the food on offer. For those with advancing dementia actually providing the choice of meals already plated (rather than the picture of a meal) may be a better way of providing choice as it is more easily recognised and has led to improved intake (Desai et al., 2007).

Life story / Talking Mats

Life story is a communication activity in which the person with dementia and the people caring for them gather and review past life experiences to build a personal biography (Dementia UK, 2017). It is possible to apply the activity to mealtimes by gathering past food preferences and mealtime routine although this is not what it is specifically designed for. Other communication aids include 'Talking Mats', which has a dementia and mealtime-specific resource to help identify choices of food and the preferred setting to eat (Talking Mats, 2017). Life story work or using communication aids such as Talking Mats (which are used outside of the mealtime setting) can help carers build a closer relationship with the person living with dementia. Research into their effectiveness for improving nutritional intake is required.

Meal service style

An interesting study in which carers ate their meals with care home residents with advanced dementia found that the increased social interaction helped the carers become more aware of individual residents' likes, dislikes and preferences. The residents with dementia were also more inclined to reveal personal life stories (Charras and Frémontier, 2010).

A further study changed the way food was served to care home residents with dementia. Here a cafeteria style with waitress service was adopted and involved showing residents all the food available and allowing them to choose the foods and quantity they desired, and this led to increased food intake (Desai *et al.*, 2007). These two studies are discussed in more detail under 'Lunch' and 'Dinner' in the 'Modifying meal patterns and serving style' section that follows below.

Modifying tableware

The previous chapter on increasing independence at mealtimes discussed modifications to the tableware, which usually involved providing high contrast to plates or adapted cutlery to support self-feeding abilities. However, in this chapter on supporting preferences, the size of the plate and the portion of food provided on the plate are the important elements, both of which may affect the amount of food consumed.

Plate size

Having a large dinner plate with a large portion size of food may be off-putting to someone with a small appetite or someone who gets full quickly, as people with dementia tend to experience. Serving large portions on large plates may be a bad idea, while serving a normal portion on a large plate may actually provide additional benefits in that more food may be consumed.

The 'Delboeuf illusion' demonstrated that we perceive a difference in size between two identical circles when one is surrounded by a much larger circle and the other one is surrounded by only a slightly larger circle (Van Ittersum and Wansink, 2012). The use of this interesting visual perception can be applied to the use of plates and serving sizes and may be particularly useful for those with small appetites. For example serving a normal portion size of food on a larger plate can make the portion seem smaller than it actually is; or if you think of it from the other way around, serving the normal portion size on a smaller plate (filling a plate with food) may make the portion seem larger than it actually is.

It may still be important that the food on the plate has a colour contrast from the rest of the plate (as discussed in Chapter 4) but this should be assessed rather than assumed. Practically this means that providing a larger plate that also contrasts with the food may make the serving size appear smaller, which may benefit those with smaller appetites or loss of vision and those who often do not finish their meals. The aim is to encourage consumption of food, and modifying tableware in this instance may provide one way to do this. Unfortunately this has not been evaluated in dementia but may provide an additional non-invasive intervention. It is worth noting that using smaller plates to serve food to those with a small appetite may actually cause underserving of portion sizes by carers – leading to a reduction in food consumed.

This type of intervention should mainly be useful for those with small appetites; however, modifying tableware can also be tried for those who have a tendency to consume sweet foods. It may be worth trialling a large plate with a normal portion size for main meals and a small bowl for pudding or sweets to see if this has any effect on consumption of these foods. The aim of course is to try to increase intake from the large plate while decreasing intake from the small bowl. There is no guarantee this will have any effect but as long as overall food consumption does not decreasing this can be trialled.

Plate warmers

A common reduced mealtime ability related to preferences with eating and drinking is 'slow eating or prolonged mealtimes'. If someone living with dementia is taking an hour to eat their food there are both nutrition and safety implications to be considered. For example the swallow can fatigue over that length of time, increasing risk of aspiration, so if the person has a swallowing difficulty this should be closely monitored. If food is going cold after 15 minutes then the person is less likely to eat and this may compromise their nutritional intake. Some may argue that the person with dementia may *choose* to spend an hour eating. If they consume all of their food then this is a fine assumption. In this instance using a plate warmer or a similar piece of equipment will help keep the food warmer for longer and we would assume nicer to eat.

If on the other hand the person does struggle to consume their food and is gradually losing weight then as a carer you have to assume that they are not choosing to spend an hour eating their food or indeed choosing to become malnourished. It does not matter how long someone takes to eat and certainly they should be allowed up to an hour, although time constraints placed on carers in care homes can often rush this allowance. What really matters is the support provided to them during their mealtime. Plate warmers can still be used in this instance; however, more assistance will be needed during an extended eating time.

Modifying meal patterns and serving styles

In free-living healthy populations the intake of food portion size and associated energy and micronutrients tends to increase over the day, peaking at dinner time. In some older adults this pattern may change and the main meal is consumed slightly earlier in the day. For people with dementia living in long-term care or when admitted into acute care the main meal is often served at lunchtime, and this may be the same for the home setting especially if paid carers are visiting to provide assistance with meals. Both the traditional meal pattern of increasing size throughout the day or providing the majority of food at lunchtime may be detrimental to a certain group of people living with dementia. Those with a lower BMI or who experience behavioural symptoms at mealtimes may benefit the most from a change in these traditional meal patterns. Interventions should focus on breakfast, additional snacks or small regular meals to increase nutritional intake; we discuss each one of these below.

Breakfast

Anecdotally carers often report that breakfast is the most consistently consumed meal during the day, especially in care home residents with dementia (Dyer and Greenwood, 2001), while it is also the meal least often refused (Young and Greenwood, 2001). If people with dementia are more likely to consistently consume their breakfast compared to other meals then breakfast provides an opportunity for nutritional intervention.

This theory was tested and the results confirmed what is often seen in practice in that the intake of food and drink at breakfast is less erratic than at other mealtimes, meaning more people were more likely to eat more of the food provided at breakfast (Young and Greenwood, 2001). This however highlights an issue with the current provision of food in care settings at breakfast, where it often consists of cereal or toast, partly owing to the lower costs of these ingredients and also the fact that no catering staff are required to prepare the food. The breakfast meal is often lower in energy (calories), fat and protein compared to lunch or dinner meals, while carbohydrate intakes are similar across all three mealtimes (Dyer and Greenwood, 2001).

The addition of fat and protein to increase overall energy provided at breakfast is often implemented in the form of food fortification, by using full-fat milk (fat) and adding milk powder (protein) to milk served on cereal or in drinks.

The other option is to provide a cooked meal at breakfast, for example eggs, beans, toast, tomatoes and so on, which would have a similar nutrient profile to the lunch meals usually served. This type of intervention requires a change in the meal pattern. Commonly lunch is the main meal of the day and when the most calories and nutrients are available to be consumed. If however someone consistently consumes breakfast while eating only very small amounts at lunch, they will be missing out on this main opportunity to consume calories and nutrients. Of course if someone is not consuming their meal at lunch then there may be many factors that contribute to this, as discussed throughout Chapters 4 to 11. For example the environment at the lunch meal may not be supportive for their current level of mealtime abilities, or reduced eating abilities may impact on food consumed. Providing a cooked meal at breakfast will therefore also increase the eating abilities needed to self-feed. This is an interesting point, as although research indicates breakfast is the most consistently consumed meal (Young and Greenwood, 2001) we do not know why this is. We have to consider whether this is due to breakfast being relatively easy to eat. For example cereal is served in a bowl and only a spoon is required to eat it, or toast can be eaten using just hands. Certainly a cooked breakfast can be served as a finger food option as sausages, boiled eggs, toast, hash browns and so on can all be easily manipulated by hand. In a care home fewer staff may be available to assist at breakfast if a cooked version is provided which could impact on the success of the cooked breakfast intervention, while a home carer may not need to worry about these issues. As breakfast is the meal provided following the longest duration between eating, and people with dementia may experience satiety quicker, this may also be a factor for the more consistent intakes observed, where hunger levels are highest at breakfast compared to lunch or dinner.

Whether choosing to fortify food at breakfast or providing a cooked meal, a key point to consider is that this intervention may be most suited to those who eat little at lunch and/or are at risk of malnutrition. There will always be individual differences, hence it is important to assess and monitor the intervention used and not use a blanket approach to change everyone's breakfast. For example for someone who has reduced abilities to use a knife and fork, introducing a cooked breakfast may cause them to eat less. It may be more beneficial to fortify their breakfast cereal, which is easier for them to consume, and also trial the use of cooked breakfast finger foods to see if this is acceptable.

IN SUMMARY

Breakfast is usually the most consistently consumed meal in care home residents with dementia, particularly those with a low BMI, advanced dementia and at higher risk of malnutrition. This may be due to the relative ease of consuming one or two items of traditional breakfast foods and/or the decreased satiety levels at breakfast, meaning hunger levels are higher. Providing more calories and nutrients at breakfast via cooked meals or fortified foods is therefore a potential nutritional intervention. The success of the intervention will need to be tailored to the person as taste preferences, eating abilities and carer assistance can all impact the amount of food consumed.

Lunch

Sometimes the most energy-dense meal is the one least consumed and unfortunately this is often lunch. These meals are provided in dining environments where some people with dementia find it harder to eat owing to excess stimuli. Additionally they may already be feeling full, perhaps from a mid-morning snack or supplement, or they have their own individual preferences which have not been accounted for. Simply they may like to eat their main meal in the evening or as a large brunch, preferring not to have lunch. Midday is traditionally thought of as the best time to maximise food intake as more staff are around and cognitive abilities are better; however, cognitive skills may be more enhanced at other times of the day (Young *et al.*, 2001). Furthermore providing a variety of foods at one time can present a challenge to some people with reduced mealtime abilities or those who are sensitive to overstimulation in a busy mealtime environment, increasing their agitation.

In an effort to increase the intake of food from the main mealtime, carers in a care home in France decided to 'share' their lunch meal with the residents by eating alongside them (Charras and Frémontier, 2010). This change in food service style provided some interesting insights which will be discussed below. It is worth noting that from a research perspective there was a huge selection bias as the carers volunteered to initiate the intervention, which makes its replication dependent on the same level of initiative from carers in other care homes. To add further confusion to the true beneficial outcomes of carers eating their meals with people with dementia, two other interventions were administered at the same time. Environmental changes were made to the care homes including small changes to furniture, decorations and linen, and previous to this the carers also took part in a 12-session training programme on dementia care. Indeed it was this training that prompted the carers to think of the idea to start eating meals with the residents.

Practically the intervention included sharing the lunch meal: the carers sat on the same tables, consisting of eight to nine residents, and they provided assistance to those who required it. Eighteen people with severe cognitive impairment as assessed by the Mini-Mental State Examination (MMSE) took part in this study. It was also ensured that the mealtime was 'quiet and orderly', and in line with French cultural norms a four-course meal was served (starter, main, cheese, dessert). Food was served collectively in dishes so staff and residents could serve themselves or their neighbour. For the cheese course a cheese board was passed around the table, again providing a self-service option. At the end of the meal coffee or tea was provided for staff and residents and consumed collectively. Six months after this 'sharing' of the lunch meal was implemented the residents had gained on average 3.37kg (7.4 pounds) while a control group not receiving a shared lunch meal had lost an average 2.22kg. As mentioned, large bias in the recruitment of participants means these results are not reliable but in practice it shows weight can be increased even in those with severe cognitive impairment.

Perhaps the most interesting findings to come from this study were in the observations and reports from staff following the intervention, and it is a shame these were not measured as part of the research outcomes. The findings relate directly to what mealtime dementia care should be trying to achieve, which is an improvement in the way mealtimes are provided for people living with dementia. These findings are not robust from a research point of view but they are very poignant and worthy of inclusion here.

- **Independence** – Residents were seen eating independently again, with other residents trying to pick up their cutlery to eat by themselves. Residents seemed happy to help set and clear the table including sweeping after the meal. As much as possible residents served themselves the portion size of food they wanted with some taking or asking for seconds.

- **Social interactions** – Carer interactions with residents increased with carers emphasising that they became more aware of individual residents' likes, dislikes and preferences. Residents helped each other at the meals with some reminiscing and being more inclined to reveal personal life stories.

- **Meal behaviours** – Residents known to walk during meals tended to stay seated for longer or sometimes sat through the entire meal, while others who often expressed concerns about paying for meals or asking for the bill did not do this when meals were shared.

- **Staff job satisfaction** – Carers reported increased satisfaction with the shared meal conditions and were observed staying a bit longer than their shift and greeting residents before going, allowing additional time for meals and reminiscing about pleasant parts of the meal. Carers reported satisfaction that they were not only providing physical care but had done something useful at the end of their day's work. It is a shame job satisfaction is not used more as an outcome in research of this kind.

- **Organisational** – Interestingly carers considered wearing uniforms at mealtimes an institutional barrier to creating the homelike environment they were trying to achieve. Carers also provided first-hand feedback directly to the catering team on the food provided, which they felt improved during the study and also helped them understand why some residents did not eat certain meals. The length of shared meals was between one and one and a half hours.

IN SUMMARY

The simplicity of this piece of research is that the main intervention was eating meals with people with dementia. The confounding factors include environmental changes to make the dining room more homelike, training of carers and clear bias in who the interventions were chosen for. Regardless of this these multicomponent interventions are commonly used in reality and really should be praised. The effects from this simple intervention can be vast and although not all care homes could adopt this approach it surely must be worth considering for some. Whether the sharing of meals increased food intake via increased social interactions, improved cueing to eat and drink, better assistance by carers, more food and portion size choice (from serving their own food) or a decrease in meal behaviours is really unknown. What is clear is that sharing meals in this instance improved all of these factors, which can ensure adequate nutrition being consumed, and provided improved socialisation.

Dinner

Research studies indicate that both service-style adaptation, as mentioned in the study from France at lunchtimes above, and adaptations to the actual food served may enhance food intake at dinner time. Both of these interventions will be considered in this section on dinner, which is described here as the evening meal.

ADAPTING THE FOOD PROVIDED

Research conducted in care homes has indicated that 88 per cent of residents with dementia do not meet their energy (calorie) requirements, with 37 per cent of these also not meeting protein requirements (Young and Greenwood, 2001). This study highlighted that decreased intakes at dinner contributed to this by providing the lowest energy consumption of all three main meals. It was also more apparent in residents with advanced dementia displaying behavioural symptoms and confusion, and with a lower BMI. These particular residents consumed the largest percentage of their energy intake at breakfast and the least at dinner.

The authors suggested that it was the shift in circadian eating patterns that caused residents to eat more at breakfast than at dinner. In other words they thought that cognitive skills were reduced later in the day and that 'sundowning' played a significant role in decreased food intake around this time. It needs to be pointed out that the authors did not look at any changes in mealtime abilities between breakfast and dinner. The decreased intakes at dinner observed could in part be due to the environment, where eating abilities were not fully supported at this evening meal, causing the reduced intake that was observed. This highlights a need to assess mealtime abilities at dinner time in addition to lunchtime if food intakes are observed to be inadequate at the evening meal.

Another reason for decreased intake may be the type of food served at dinner, while the 'fast' overnight may lead to more hunger at breakfast. People with dementia tend to reach satiety early so a long period of not eating at night may have contributed to increased intakes at breakfast rather than dinner. This does not change the fact that dinner may be a poorly consumed meal, so the authors looked at interventions to increase calorie intake.

In one of the very few randomised controlled trials in people living with dementia where normal food was the only intervention, the same authors replaced the care home residents' traditional evening meal with a high-carbohydrate meal (Young et al., 2005). This meal would consist of breakfast foods (cereal and milk) but also included boiled eggs, muffins, bread and jam and so on. The intervention meal provided the same amount of energy and protein as the care home's traditional evening meal but supplied more carbohydrate and less fat. Twenty out of the thirty-two residents increased their intake but interestingly the residents in whom the intervention was most effective were those with greater cognitive impairment (advanced dementia), more motor problems, increased disengagement and a preference for carbohydrate foods. Mealtime abilities were not assessed in this study but it is likely that motor problems as the authors put it will impact on eating ability as will disengagement. Furthermore as these individuals also had advanced dementia then it is likely the level of mealtime abilities were lower.

As the majority of people increased their intake we have to ask whether this means that providing high-carbohydrate foods to people with advanced dementia and reduced mealtime abilities is a suitable intervention at dinner time. Interestingly the choice of high-carbohydrate intervention foods included things like cereal, hard boiled eggs, slices of bread and jam, half a muffin, slices of fruit and cheese and bananas, all of which are suitable finger foods and/or require fewer eating abilities to consume, as well as being very similar to breakfast foods. The authors' conclusion from the study at the time was that there can be a shift in preference for high-carbohydrate foods; therefore providing these foods increases intake.

Three years later however the same authors revisited this advice and concluded that it was more likely that the food provided was easier to consume, which led to increased intake, rather than it being solely because it was carbohydrate based (Smith and Greenwood, 2008). If there was ever a study that highlighted the importance of providing food and the means to consume food at the correct level of eating ability for the individual, this this was surely it. It is a shame that the authors did not measure this mealtime ability element to prove this point, though. A final important point is that providing more choice at the evening meal, regardless of its carbohydrate content, may also have had a significant impact on the amount of food consumed.

The study showed that by simply serving breakfast food at dinner time intake can also be increased. Therefore breakfast foods could provide a useful short-term intervention for increasing food intake. While doing this, efforts can be concentrated on working out what foods are best suited for people who are not consuming their traditional evening meal. This intervention may be particularly useful and perhaps should be targeted in those with advancing dementia and reduced mealtime abilities, and/or who are experiencing more behavioural symptoms.

ADAPTING THE SERVING STYLE

The research discussed above suggests that adapting the food provided at dinner time, with an emphasis on more finger food choices and possibly a higher carbohydrate consumption, may enhance food intake, especially in individuals with more advanced dementia. Further research in care homes also highlights that you may not need to change the type of food provided to increase intake if you change the way it is served. Adopting a cafeteria style with waitress service versus a traditional tray delivery service led to increased consumption at all meals and a statistically significant increase in carbohydrate consumption: bread, potato and pasta at the dinner (evening) meal (Desai et al., 2007). The evening meal in this case was the main meal of the day. Importantly this change in service was once again most beneficial to those with a low BMI and increased cognitive impairment while those with a higher BMI did not change their intake significantly. Practically the cafeteria style with waitress service involved showing residents all the food available and allowing them to choose the foods and quantity of what they desired. This simple change in the way food is delivered is thought to increase intake through the following means:

- improved plate presentation

- improved temperature of the meal

- increased food choice at the time of service

- portion size flexibility.

All of this can also be achieved through more traditional pre-plated food service delivery but the server would have to know the likes, dislikes and preferences for each person before plating the food. This of course can be very difficult to achieve in a group care setting; therefore to help gain an understanding of individual preferences this style of service may be extremely useful in this context.

There is one more very important aspect that a more personalised service style provides that is much harder to measure, and this is social interaction. The greater social interaction between staff serving and the person with dementia could be an essential factor in helping to achieve increased food and fluid intake. Indeed the authors of this study commented that the new service style likely allowed more time for other carers to focus on facilitating food intake rather than worrying about serving food and getting portion sizes correct (Desai *et al.*, 2007).

Limitations of these findings include the fact that residents in this care home could eat independently and had no swallowing difficulties. Whether this change in food service could be effective in those with reduced mealtime abilities is unknown and it is a shame mealtime abilities were not measured. Furthermore, at the same time the style of food service was changed, there were also environmental changes with a shift from an institutional appearance to more homelike setting, which may also have improved intake. From an organisational point of view in a care home, if this type of food service was to be adopted it is worth noting that it is more likely to benefit those at higher risk of malnutrition (low BMI), which is of course who the intervention is typically aimed at. As an example a volunteer in a care home setting could be tasked with showing and serving the food while trained care assistants are used to provide additional support. In addition care providers found this type of service resulted in reduced food wastage (Desai *et al.*, 2007).

Summary of modifying meal patterns and serving style

What seems clear from the research on changing meal patterns, serving styles and adapting the type of food available is that a multicomponent intervention seems to produce the best results. Both studies that adapted the serving styles for the main meals served at either lunch (Charras and Frémontier, 2010) or dinner (Desai *et al.*, 2007) also changed the environment or provided training to carers. Even the study that adapted the type of food to make it predominant in carbohydrate intake inadvertently created more finger food options (Young *et al.*, 2005). In the previous chapter (4) on supporting independence and eating abilities multicomponent research enhanced both lighting and colour contrast at the same time (Brush *et al.*, 2012). All of these multicomponent interventions found an improved food intake as well as improvements in mealtime abilities and meal behaviours. A multicomponent strategy in relation to mealtime dementia care is perhaps the most effective means of improving the nutritional care of people living with dementia and is what this book advocates. Table 6.1 summarises the practical application of the research evidence discussed in this section.

Table 6.1: Modifying meal patterns and serving styles to enhance nutritional intake

Mealtime	Potential issues	Potential changes
Breakfast	Tends to be the most consistently consumed meal but also tends to provide the least nutrients	Utilise consistent intakes by fortifying foods and/or making breakfast a main meal more often
Lunch (afternoon)	Usually the main meal but an unsupportive lunchtime environment can affect mealtime abilities and intake	Ensure a supportive mealtime environment (see Chapters 10 and 11) and increase socialisation via sharing meals or assisting with self-service styles to enhance mealtime abilities
Dinner (evening)	Can be the worst consumed meal of the day for some	Provide more choice including finger food options and even repeat breakfast food options to increase food intake

Food First advice

Food First advice is based around the premise of providing normal food as the first line of treatment for people who are at risk of malnutrition. This may sound a bit odd to those who are not employed carers or health professionals. Unfortunately over the last decade or more there has been a gradual medicalisation of food where oral nutrition supplements (ONS) rather than real food are provided as a means to increase nutritional intake. The companies that provide these supplements are intricately linked in malnutrition policy and with organisations providing advice to carers such as large national charities. However, this book is not the place for a discussion of these issues. There are plenty of excellent resources that provide Food First advice for people with dementia such as the Caroline Walker Trust (Crawley and Hocking, 2011). Information on Food First advice can also be provided by dietitians and there are freely available resources linked to NHS trusts' dietetic departments such as the one by Essex Partnership University NHS Foundation Trust (EPUT, 2017). An entire book can be written on providing Food First advice to people with dementia, therefore in this section a few key practical points will be briefly discussed concerning the main three Food First treatments of:

1. food fortification

2. snacks

3. nourishing drinks.

Food fortification

One study found that despite food to meet older people's nutritional requirements being available in care settings, intakes are often below those needed to prevent weight loss (Leslie *et al.*, 2013). The use of food fortification is one way to enrich food to lessen weight loss, and their study shows it can be successful even in older adults who have a BMI of below 18.5kg/m^2, in the short term at least. Fortifying food is an economical and simple way of increasing the density of energy (calories) and macronutrients (fat, carbohydrate and protein) provided without increasing portion size, it may be particularly useful for those with small appetites. The increase in fat can be the main contributing factor to increasing weight and BMI when fortification is used (Leslie *et al.*, 2013). Compared to providing ONS, less taste fatigue may be seen when normal food is fortified. Food also helps to maintain normal eating patterns and eating abilities rather than reliance on a pre-prepared nutrition supplement drink, often consumed from a plastic bottle.

One of the most important and yet probably overlooked aspect of fortification is accommodating the person's tastes and preferences for which fortification methods are used. Traditionally dairy sources such as butter, cream, full-fat milk or milk powder are used and are common food sources in a British diet. Adding butter or cream to all the food you wish to fortify, however, is likely to be unpalatable for many and may lead to taste fatigue. With the multicultural society in Britain especially in urban areas more thought should be applied to fortification choices. The use of a range of oils (olive, rapeseed, sesame, etc.) at 120 calories per tablespoon provides an excellent alternative to cream for example and may be more acceptable to those who have not traditionally consumed lots of dairy products. Similarly fortification methods can also be used to enhance the flavour of foods. Creating a pesto or pistou using oil, herbs, cheese and nuts provides additional flavour and fortification to meals and traditionally works well with pasta or when added to soups. Care staff need to work closely with the catering and management team to identify potential food fortification ideas specific to the person rather than just adding butter and cream to everything. As with all nutritional interventions in dementia, evaluating the use of food fortification requires a lot more robust research and often will need to be used in combination with other interventions if any effective outcomes are to be achieved.

If dietary assessment as usually conducted by a dietitian reveals inadequate intakes of calories and protein from normal food intake then preventing protein-energy malnutrition often becomes the aim of treatment. Interventions can include eating smaller regular meals every five hours with a source of protein (e.g. 15g) that is liked at each meal. Simple ways to include additional protein along with energy can include adding cheese on toast at breakfast rather than jam, adding egg into rice to create a stir-fried egg rice, trying protein bars or granola/nut/seed bars or cheese and crackers as snacks, or having ice-cream for pudding. Examples of other effective, typical food fortification strategies used by carers include adding whey protein powder to soups (Shatenstein et al., 2008).

Snacks

When looking at snacks as part of a daily meal pattern they can be seen as an 'all or none' phenomenon with some people relying on snacks to maintain their nutrition status while others don't consume any (Young and Greenwood, 2001). Snack foods are often entirely consumed, unlike meals, highlighting that if a nutritious snack is provided it can contribute greatly to meeting nutritional requirements. Interestingly those with a lower BMI often consume very similar amounts of breakfast compared to those with a higher BMI but consume less at lunch and dinner (Young and Greenwood, 2001). These people do however consume a larger percentage of their intake from snacks, indicating a 'little and often' approach with smaller meals, but regular nutritious snacks can help maintain overall nutrition intake. Providing little and often is a common, practical and useful approach but it is also important to optimise nutritional intake when the person is alert or having a 'better day'.

Snacks can increase food and fluid intake and increase body weight. If offering between-meal snacks it is important these do not affect the intake at main meals as some research has shown (Simmons, Zhuo and Keeler, 2010). If snacks do decrease mealtime intake close monitoring will be needed to determine if overall the person is eating less than before the snacks were introduced. A loss of weight is an indication that this is the case. Snacks can be as effective or more effective and cost less than prescribed oral nutrition supplements and also result in lower refusal rates and less carer time to promote consumption (Simmons *et al.*, 2010). A change in the serving style and the way snacks are presented and offered may provide a longer-lasting impact on improving nutritional intake (Desai *et al.*, 2007). Practical aspects of snack delivery will make the effectiveness of a snack intervention more effective. Here are some ideas:

- If possible group people together in groups of four when administering the snacks to help with social interaction; this also means that if carer assistance is needed it can be provided to several people at once.

- A good time for a snack period is 15 to 20 minutes, with carer assistance if needed to encourage individuals to eat independently.

- Snacks are best delivered between meals but not too close to a mealtime and are probably better provided sooner after a mealtime than nearer the next mealtime.

- A variety of snacks should be available and may be presented on a snack cart or displayed attractively so the visual stimulation can promote appetite.

- Snacks can be of normal calorific value, around 100kcals (fruit, fruit juice, yoghurt, biscuit, etc.), or high energy, around 250kcals (croissant, ice-cream, cake, cheese and biscuits, etc.), depending on the amount of additional calories and nutrition that needs to be provided.

- It is important both to monitor the intake of snacks, whether someone needs assistance and the best time of day snacks are accepted, and to discover preferences for snacks (recorded in their care plan). This takes more time at the start but saves time in the long run.

- Most snacks are also useful finger foods and as such require fewer eating abilities to consume.

- Mealtime abilities can affect the consumption of snacks. Mealtime assessment tools such as the dementia mealtime assessment tool (DMAT, 2017) can be used to help evaluate the mealtime abilities needed to consume the snacks and highlight potential swallowing difficulties to further individualise the support offered.

- If the snacks are refused more often than consumed then other interventions should be trialled, and/or better prompting and/or delivery of snacks by carers should be evaluated.

- If when providing snacks someone still does not increase intake look for other interventions and consult with a dietitian to assess overall nutritional intake.

Nourishing drinks

It can often be easier to consume nutrition in a liquid rather than a solid form. This is especially true for those who have small appetites, become full quickly, tire during mealtimes or have reduced eating abilities. Nourishing drinks include homemade or pre-bought milkshakes, smoothies, soups or drinks made from a powdered form such as protein powders or other specifically designed nutritional powdered drinks. There really are no rules when making a nourishing drink; the aim is to provide a good source of calories and protein along with some essential vitamins and minerals in an accepted form. Nourishing drinks can be administered in the same way as snacks, described previously, and can also be offered as a meal replacement if a meal is missed or only a small amount is eaten. Examples of nourishing drinks can be provided by a dietitian or found by searching the useful Food First resources on NHS websites.

Healthy eating

It is worth remembering that, as dementia progresses, the importance of healthy eating is outweighed by the importance of consuming enough calories to prevent significant weight loss. Healthy eating is also outweighed by someone's preferences for their quality of life and enjoyment. If after attempting many different ways to provide a variety of food options all someone wants to eat is cornflakes with chocolate milk buttons then so be it. This preferred intake is still far superior to struggling to get them to eat food they do not want to, as apart from them not eating it this will also cause increased stress for them and most likely the carer too. Alibhai *et al.*'s (2005) research suggests eating favourite foods may even improve outcomes such as increased weight and appetite. This research also indicates that dietary restrictions for health reasons, for example a low-salt diet for high blood pressure or a low-sugar diet for diabetes, may no longer be medically indicated and can increase risk of weight loss. In addition it may contribute to poor appetite as the food does not taste good (ADA, 2005). In the instance of weight loss or reduced nutritional intake a dietitian should be consulted as to the continued appropriateness of any diets. Indeed a position statement from the American Dietetic Association suggests that liberalisation of prescribed diets can help enhance quality of life and nutritional status in older adults in long-term care (ADA, 2005).

Oral nutrition supplements

The concept of oral nutrition supplements (ONS) sounds like a great idea on paper. ONS are a 'nutritionally complete' drink of which you consume two to three every day to provide all your nutritional needs, although this may not include your total energy (calorie) requirements. The limited research into their use in dementia however indicates that temporary use of ONS can be both beneficial and detrimental to nutritional intake and body weight in people living with dementia (Parrott, Young and Greenwood, 2006).

To be effective ONS must be consumed. Although there are several practical ways to increase compliance and consumption of ONS they all require additional staff resources which are frequently lacking in dementia care. Certainly if the correct level of assistance is provided then providing snacks or oral food may be just as or more effective and cost less than providing ONS (Simmons *et al.*, 2010).

Additionally the current screening tools used in the assessment for prescription of ONS such as the Malnutrition Universal Screening Tool (MUST) may not be specific enough to assess the nutritional complexities in people with dementia. Those identified as at risk of malnutrition by low BMI (<20kg/m^2) and/or with advanced dementia may not respond to ONS as an effective intervention (Hanson *et al.*, 2011).

There is a need to assess the precursors to decreased nutritional intake and weight loss, such as reduced mealtime abilities (Allen, Methven and Gosney, 2013), and intervene at this stage.

As the use of ONS in dementia has undergone the most research and outcomes of effectiveness are still not clear (Hanson *et al.*, 2011), we should remember they may have both positive and negative effects on health outcomes and as such should always involve a dietitian as part of a treatment strategy. A short-term increase in energy intake does not seem to be matched by any long-term weight maintenance or any improvement in dementia-related symptoms. Indeed recommendations for dietitians include using practical, achievable strategies that focus on Food First advice and adapting eating environments to promote oral intake for people living with dementia (Jansen *et al.*, 2015).

This chapter discusses preferences with eating and drinking, and there is no research indicating that people with dementia have a preference for ONS over traditional food. Most likely ONS would not be their preferred choice to increase nutrition and we should remember this when deciding on appropriate interventions to increase nutritional intake. People living with dementia rely more on sensory cues and familiarity of foods along with social interaction at mealtimes. Providing food in the form of ONS will take away many of these important mealtime aspects. Certainly limited evidence exists that in people with dementia who had a low BMI (and the people who are usually targeted for ONS) there was actually a decrease in their intake of habitual (normal) food when provided with ONS (Young *et al.*, 2004). The provision of ONS did not lead to enhanced nutritional intake overall either and when the ONS were stopped their habitual food intake did not return (Parrott *et al.*, 2006).

Often the nutritional pathways for managing malnutrition recommend the use of ONS, and malnutrition charities are aligned with nutritional supplement companies to promote this message. It is important for the carer to be aware that most ONS research trials in people with dementia have focused on those at risk of malnutrition or who are normally nourished. The effectiveness of ONS in people with dementia who are already malnourished is not fully known and may be detrimental to some (Prince *et al.*, 2014).

Much can be written on this subject but it is not relevant for the purpose of this book; however for further information and for practical advice on using ONS in dementia, additional articles are freely available (Martin, 2017).

Stimulate senses

The senses of smell and taste are lost as we all get older, and these losses can be heightened in people living with dementia. The loss of these important senses can contribute to poor appetite, changes in food choice (which may be inappropriate for nutritional quality), decreased nutritional intake and enjoyment of food (Schiffman and Graham, 2000). The aromas and flavours of food can also be powerful in evoking memories (Schiffman, 1983). Perhaps as these senses are lost the recognition of culturally preferred food becomes diminished in people with dementia.

Quite often the interventions used to increase the nutritional intake of people who may be experiencing sensory losses do not take these factors into account. Traditional nutritional interventions to increase nutritional content such as food fortification, eating little and often or using oral nutrition supplements do not compensate for these sensory losses. Therefore to provide individuals with food they prefer, taste adaptations to the foods can be made to enhance their sensory inputs.

Taste preferences

Taste preferences change with age and are commonly seen in people living with dementia, some of whom have a tendency for more sweet-tasting foods. Often the sense of taste is not completely absent (the medical term for this is ageusia) but may be reduced (hypogeusia) or distorted (dysgeusia). For example with dysgeusia this distorted taste could include sensing bitter or metallic tastes when eating foods (Schiffman and Graham, 2000). Taste thresholds for amino acids (protein), sweeteners and sodium chloride (salt) can be two-and-a-half times higher in the elderly compared to younger people (Schiffman, 1983). This means in practice the person with dementia may consume excess sugar and prefer sweet foods or find food is bland as they cannot detect the sweetness or salt flavours in their foods. An increased threshold for sweetness may also mean someone will prefer to eat sweet foods, leading to lower intakes of protein and micronutrients (vitamins and minerals). Increased threshold for salt may mean too that foods such as meat, fish, poultry, vegetables, cereal and grains have less taste and are not eaten. These negative influences of taste changes will possibly mean using interventions that provide more salty food and adapting foods to enhance their natural sweetness or making them taste sweeter.

PREFERENCE FOR SWEET FOODS

Preference for sweet foods can mean puddings and snacks become main food intakes and savoury dishes including meat and vegetables are eaten less. Eating dessert before the rest of the meal was a frequent observation in one mealtime-based study on people with dementia (Durnbaugh et al., 1996). With some simple modifications to the savoury meals, however, sweetness can be provided, for example by adding prunes or apricots to meat dishes, honey-glazing gammon with pineapple, using apple or cranberry sauce and so on. Other adaptations can include sweeter-tasting vegetables (e.g. sweet potato, sweetcorn), sweet sauces or extra sugar in gravies provided with meat, and adding sugar in the cooking of vegetables or protein sources.

Additionally an increased taste threshold for amino acids (protein) may provide a positive effect as protein powders may be added to foods, especially sweet foods, without a noticeable change in taste. The range of protein powders available nowadays are vast and include those derived from plants and grains rather than the typical whey-based powders. This in itself provides additional interventions. For example a pea protein powder would work extremely well in a pea-based soup. This type of soup is naturally slightly sweet, and ham and Parmesan can be used to add salty flavour and additional protein. Using easily accessible and practical techniques such as this is currently a hugely under-researched and under-appreciated part of potential nutrition-based interventions. Actual evidence on the effectiveness of these suggested flavour enhancements in improving food intake or preference for these foods (over other foods) would be very welcome.

PRACTICAL WAYS TO STIMULATE THE SENSE OF TASTE

Alternating between the different foods on the plate so every mouthful is different from the last may help enhance the flavours in the meal and increase intake. The variety of textures between the meat and vegetables may also slightly compensate for a loss of taste, as will the action of chewing (Schiffman, 1983). Indeed this provides another good reason why soft or puréed food should not be mixed together as every mouthful will taste the same. The person will encounter sensory adaptation to the meal as the flavour from the first mouthful will diminish with successive mouthfuls. The addition of condiments to meals may also provide an additional flavour stimulus.

Smell preferences

Taste and smell are linked, with 70 per cent of our taste coming from aromas detected by our nose. The sense of smell can be more impacted by age than taste alone, meaning the smell of food may need to be stronger for an older person to detect it (Schiffman, 1983). For someone with dementia who perhaps does not fully recognise all of the food in front of them, having even less ability to detect smells from foods means these useful cues are lost. The only benefit of this is that unpleasant smells too will be less detected. The sense of smell may also affect appetite where pleasant aromas increase appetite while no sense or lack of sense of smell may actually decrease appetite. The reduction in smell and taste means catering for people with dementia needs more thought, and several practical options are available to enhance the smell of foods to stimulate the sense of smell.

FLAVOUR-ENHANCED FOOD

Stronger-flavoured foods and the use of commercial flavour enhancements can be used to 'amplify' the aromas of foods. Commercial flavours can be added to food when cooking or at the table and these simply contain odorous compounds but no taste flavours like salt or sweeteners. It's important to note that these flavour enhancement techniques are different to simply adding more spices, herbs or salt. Adding extra flavours such as these will provide different and more varied odours and tastes but will not provide the increase in one specific intense flavour, for example using a beef flavour in beef stock. Benefits of flavour-enhanced food can include improved palatability, improved intake and increased saliva although no statistically significant increases in calorie or nutrient intake have been detected (Schiffman and Graham, 2000). Studies have shown that older people, although not those living with dementia, prefer foods that have had their flavour enhanced and that food intake can be increased in clinical settings (Schiffman and Warwick, 1993). When using six powdered flavours (roast beef, ham, bacon, beef, maple, cheese) to enhance certain meals and foods (soups, gravies, eggs, vegetables, stews, sauces, oatmeal, macaroni) in a group of older people an increased food intake was recorded from the flavour-enhanced foods and an increase in grip strength was shown, although this was likely not clinically significant (Schiffman and Warwick, 1993). The application and effectiveness of these interventions in people living with dementia and/or experiencing weight loss is not known but does provide a practical way to increase sensory input at mealtimes.

FOOD AROMAS

Freshly baked bread, toast, brewing coffee, baked cakes or pies or even frying bacon all present a form of sensory stimulation involving smell. Specific smells such as these or simply the smell of whatever is being cooked at the mealtimes may help stimulate the person with dementia to eat. Whatever option is chosen to trial it is important to monitor any effects, and if increasing these food aromas in a care home be aware that certain smells may not be liked by everyone. Importantly these types of food aroma interventions will only be effective in those who have a reduced ability to smell, which is termed hyposmia. If no smells can be detected, such as when someone has anosmia, then this type of intervention will not be effective (Schiffman, 1983). There are clever devices that release fragrances of food before and during mealtimes that can be substituted for 'real food' smells in an attempt to stimulate appetite.[1] Simple 'scent cards' are also available although perhaps these are more appropriate for evoking memories of foods rather than stimulating appetite.

Texture of foods

Providing foods with additional stimuli in the form of different textures may partially compensate for loss of taste and smell (Schiffman, 1983). Research has indicated that diversity of food texture is valued by those with a loss of smell (anosmia) (Alibhai et al., 2005). Indeed if taste and smell are both lost or diminished significantly then the only sensation left from having food in the mouth will come from its texture and also its temperature. Try alternating temperature and taste within meals (for example, warm stewed apple with ice-cream, or curry with yoghurt) to increase sensory stimulation.

---

1   For example see http://www.myode.org/

The stimulation of senses provided by the texture of food can also include finger foods. Using finger food and therefore physically handling the food can be a very useful way of stimulating interest in it. In addition it may provide a valuable alternative to sight, smell and taste alterations and deterioration in older people with dementia.

Food manufacturers producing crisps spend a lot of time and money each year trying to perfect a crisp with the perfect crunch noise, as do some cereal companies, and hopefully this type of sensory application will transfer into meals provided for people with dementia at some point soon. In the meantime using cereals (e.g. Cornflakes or Rice Krispies), popcorn, crisps, crackers or other suitable foods may be useful in providing an extra stimulus to either initiate eating or enhance the sensory aspects of snacks or foods for people with dementia.

Food-based activities

Another way to stimulate the senses is through food-based activities, which may provide the necessary encouragement to improve eating or may evoke old memories of foods, providing a positive experience (SCIE, 2015a). There are many activities that can take place and a few ideas follow, without going into detail. Activities can include helping to prepare foods or cooking, being more involved in typical mealtime tasks or having themed social food events. For example an afternoon tea event could combine all food activities into the same day. As mentioned in the section on 'choice' the use of life story work can be focused around food to stimulate interest in food. Finally using food as part of 'cueing' techniques at a mealtime can also be useful to stimulate interest in eating. Cueing was mainly discussed in Chapter 4, and one type of cueing involved the use of conversations at mealtimes based on principles of reminiscence. In this example food would be used as the topic of conversation. The use of these food activities has been shown to improve the nutritional status of people with dementia (Vitale et al., 2009).

Summary of stimulating senses

The food being provided to a person living with dementia who experiences loss of taste and smell may mean they find that food unpalatable. This could be a reason they either do not eat the food, or restrict their variety of foods eaten. These factors can lead to decreased nutritional intake and weight loss, increasing the risk of malnutrition.

Herbs, salt and spices increase variety of flavour but do not enhance flavour itself. Specific flavour-enhanced food may be more useful as this increases the sense of smell which stimulates taste. Interestingly, using flavour enhancement to improve the sense of smell may also evoke memories and therefore may not only improve taste but additionally trigger pleasant thoughts (Schiffman and Graham, 2000). The key point to providing stimulation to the senses of taste and smell is to make the food appear more palatable and therefore more likely to be accepted. Eating food that tastes good usually makes you feel good and therefore provides psychological wellbeing and enjoyment.

From a catering perspective there can be a lot to think about when making sensory adaptations to food and drink to optimise sensory input as just described. An increase in time and effort on the part of carers and catering teams will be required to help meet the preferences of those who are not consuming enough food and nutrition. People living with dementia, particularly in care homes, often have little say on these aspects of food provision. Ensuring as much communication with a person as possible will help the carer recognise preferences with specific food and meals. This may require the use of life story work or using communication aids such as Talking Mats to identify preferences and improve the choices offered. At the very least assessing and monitoring the impact of sensory adaptation of foods on oral intake using food record charts or similar documentation will provide some indications.

Manipulating the flavour and aroma of foods to stimulate the sense of taste and smell for people with dementia and the elderly is a fascinating area of potential research and provides opportunity for food manufacturers and food scientists' involvement. Certainly a range of flavour-enhanced foods or at least easier access to commercial flavours would be a great starting point. If more emphasis was placed on interventions like this rather than the current focus on providing different flavoured oral nutrition supplements then more options for nutritious and enjoyable normal food would be available. At present this remains a future possibility and maybe it needs a champion, someone like Heston Blumenthal perhaps, to push the agenda forward. In fact there is some research starting to emerge from a group at the University of Reading (Tsikritzi et al., 2015) and we can only hope this type of research leads to something practical and usable in care settings along with the additional catering funding required to make it happen.

Finally it is worth noting that medications can have a directed impact on taste or smell by increasing the taste threshold for flavours (Schiffman and Graham, 2000). As you can imagine, the list of medications which may have these negative side effects is long. It is beyond the capacity of this book to delve into this topic and the reader is advised to consult with the appropriate healthcare professional for advice concerning medication effects on the person they care for.

Familiarity: respecting routines and tradition
Routine
A mealtime routine can relate both to someone's routine preference (for example they do not like to eat until 11am each day), but also to cultural routines at mealtimes. A change in someone's usual eating pattern may cause decreased intake to a change in routine and normality. This can commonly occur in care settings where meals are served at set times each day. If, however, someone is used to eating almost nothing during the day and consuming most of their food in the evening then it will prove challenging for them to adapt. It is thought that people with dementia tend to display higher cognitive abilities when familiarity is applied to their environment and individual preferences are met. Family members can provide information on past life habits including the types of foods and timing of meals or if this is not possible other techniques can be utilised. The use of life story work or reminiscence therapy could help make these valuable discoveries and put together a picture of the person's daily eating and drinking routines as well as likes and dislikes. It is important to remember that routines can also change in people with dementia, and if you notice a change in routine then be guided by this change and support the new routine. Just because someone has always eaten most food in the evening this does not mean it will continue to be the case. As dementia advances, it may cause changes in routines but this may also not be the case; therefore supporting the individual becomes the most important aspect rather than figuring out why the routine has changed.

Cultural routines could include eating meals in courses, like the French four-course traditional meals discussed earlier, and also link with traditional foods discussed below. Cultural or traditional norms can include all eating from one main dish or pot of food as is typical in African cultural cuisine but also seen in many traditional British and European dishes such as shepherd's pie or lasagne.

Tradition

It has been suggested that, as dementia advances, the person finds more contentment within an environment that accords with their culture and traditions (Charras and Frémontier, 2010). Surely food can be looked upon in this same context, and sometimes for those with severe dementia the familiarity of traditional food means it is the only food they consume consistently. This return to tradition may also be another reason why research (Desai *et al.*, 2007; Charras and Frémontier, 2010) has found a positive impact on food intake when the style of food service has been changed from a more modern 'pre-plated style' (like in a restaurant) to a more traditional 'family style' (serve yourself and each other). Maybe when the generation currently in their 20s is faced with dementia it will have no problem with a pre-served/packaged plate of food but for the current generation with dementia this may seem a strange concept and the social interaction at mealtimes provided by actually serving out food may be much more acceptable. For some in this current generation food served this way may be their only memory as they may not have visited restaurants and cafés that often.

Summary

Clinical and caring experience backed up by limited research evidence shows that interventions such as food fortification or using ONS can often fail to increase weight in people living with dementia. An example of this was described in a research case study where despite intensive intervention by a dietetic team applying all the usual food fortification and ONS advice, a woman with dementia continued to lose weight. However, this same woman only two weeks previously had been consuming significantly more food when she was staying at the family's country home where she was more relaxed and interested in food. When she moved back to the city her intake declined (Shatenstein *et al.*, 2008).

It is imperative therefore that a full assessment of eating abilities, the mealtime environment and individual preferences are monitored regularly. Emphasis needs to be placed on trying the many other types of interventions described in this chapter. Providing more plentiful and appropriate food choices, changing meal patterns and nutritional content such as breakfast, adapting the serving style to make the mealtime more familiar and to increase social interaction, along with additional sensory stimulation of foods – all need to be considered. This is likely even more important for those with moderate to severe dementia who are more vulnerable. Without an individualised assessment and interventions for these people even more choice and preferences can be overlooked and care may involve a 'one size fits all' approach which clearly is not person-centred care. When asked, people with dementia have indicated that feeling at home, ability to self-feed, having a varied menu and comfortable seating are all important mealtimes experiences. Unfortunately people living with dementia are either unable or did not always feel able to speak up and request their preferences with regard to meal timings, portions size or choice of meals (Milte *et al.*, 2017).

The next chapter provides a practical way to implement the interventions described here to specifically support choice and preferences with eating and drinking.

7

Practical Interventions Section 2

AUGMENTING PREFERENCES AND CHOICE AT MEALTIMES

Assessment

Table 7.1 shows section 2 of the Dementia Mealtime Assessment Tool (DMAT, 2017) as described in Chapter 3. This section focuses on assessing preferences with eating and drinking often observed in people with dementia. Carers can use the DMAT as a simple way to assess the abilities and preferences affecting mealtimes to help plan interventions based on the person's specific needs.

Table 7.1: The DMAT section 2:
Assessment of preferences with eating and drinking

Mealtime observations: Preferences with eating and drinking	Tick observed abilities		
	Not seen	Seen once	Seen repeatedly
1. Prefers sweet food or eats desserts/sweets first			
2. Only eats certain foods			
3. Eats (or drinks) too fast			
4. Mixes food together			
5. Does not eat lunch but eats breakfast and some dinner			
6. Eats very small amounts of food (or drink)			
7. Slow eating or prolonged mealtimes			

Interventions

Multicomponent interventions where the mealtime environment, style of food service and the food are all modified are complex. Approaching the interventional changes in a systematic and structured way will help carers determine what the main issues are, what works and what does not. Gather information from the person with dementia to define their preferences and choices, or if this is challenging use communication tools and/or trial and error. This is person-centred care at its best – combining caring skills, assessment tools and evidence-based interventions and applying them to the person's needs rather than the organisation's needs.

Guidance for interventions

The interventions for supporting preferences and choice to enhance food and fluid intake can be seen as a two-part response. First the carer needs to support the person to eat and this can be achieved with interventions that involve cueing; discovering more about the person's preferences; modifying table settings, tableware or meal patterns; increasing familiarity of foods offered; and stimulating the sense of smell and taste. Hopefully this is enough to improve preferences and increase the choice of foods to people living with dementia so that they consume more.

Second the carer should adapt the food using Food First advice to fortify foods and provide more snacks, small meals and nourishing drinks to optimise the nutrition in the foods eaten. There can be little point adapting the food first if the person with dementia is not eating the food. It makes more sense to spend time identifying their preferred choices and then to modify the nutritional content of that food.

General guidance for implementing interventions can be found in the parallel section in Chapter 5, while there are a few additional guidance points specific to this section:

- In general follow the order of suggested interventions related to each identified eating ability but adapt for the individual if not appropriate.

- Try to adapt the usual food by modifying the taste, smell and familiarity first before relying on Food First advice such as nourishing drinks and food fortification.

- If a significant difference in food and fluid intake is observed at different meals, for example they eat more at dinner than lunch, then use the DMAT at these two times to investigate if there are significant differences in mealtime abilities likely affecting intake.

Suggested interventions for supporting preferences and choice to enhance food and drink consumption at mealtimes

1. Prefers sweet food or eats desserts/sweets first

- IMPORTANT NOTICE: Preference for sweet foods can lead to lower intake of calories, protein, vitamins and minerals. Monitor body weight and food intake in people who prefer sweet foods and refer to a dietitian if weight is lost.

- Provide cueing:

  - Use life story work to discover more about someone's usual eating and drinking habits, routines and personal preferences (likes and dislikes). A picture menu can be used to prompt them with other food choices that are available.

- Modify table setting:

  - Try serving meals in courses (i.e. one meal at a time). Keep desserts/sweets out of sight or not on trays/trolleys. Also offer encouragement.

- Modify tableware:

  - Trial serving main meals on large plates to make the portion size look smaller in an attempt to increase intake of main meal. Then serve the pudding on small plates or bowls, making the portion seem larger and attempting to decrease intake. It is important to note that if sweet food intake decreases, non-sweet food intake must increase to prevent weight loss.

- Stimulate senses:

  - Try increasing the natural sweetness of foods and meals to help stimulate consumption; for example add honey or sugar (or sweeteners) to carrots/parsnips when roasting. Or add sweet foods to meals, for example apricots with lamb or plums with pork.

  - Increase the flavour of the meal by enhancing one predominant flavour; for example use extra beef stock/ flavour in a beef stew. This can help enhance the smell of the dish, increasing the sense of taste.

  - Try alternating temperature and taste within meals, for example warm stewed apple with ice-cream, or curry with yoghurt, to increase sensory stimulation. If taste and smell are both diminished this can be the only sensation left.

  - Trial foods and meals with heightened sensory input, for example salty, cold, sweet, sharp, carbonated, spicy and crunchy; or foods that make your tongue tingle, for example hot or chilli sauce, menthol and ginger. These stimulate the senses and encourage food consumption.

- Increase socialisation:

  - Adapting the service style may increase interest in the meal on offer and the social interaction may stimulate eating. For example provide the opportunity for the person to serve their own food, or show the food before serving it, rather than being served pre-plated food. This can also improve portion size chosen and provide increased food choice.

  - Try eating your meal with the person. Eating with company can enhance mealtime abilities owing to social interaction and taking cues to eat from others. In addition you can help keep their focus on the meal and provide appropriate assistance if required to help maintain food intake. It can also help carers become more aware of someone's likes, dislikes and preferences.

- Food First advice:

  - Focus on quality rather than quantity of food eaten. Trial food fortification techniques to increase calories and protein; for example fortify sweet foods with protein powders/milk powder. Supplementing the diet with a multivitamin tablet may also be indicated.

  - Try offering nourishing drinks as additional snacks or after meals, for example homemade milkshakes and smoothies. These types of foods may suit the person's sweet taste preferences.

  - Think 'little and often'. Provide regular small and nutrient-dense meals, snacks, nourishing drinks or finger foods (along with sips of fluid) throughout the day rather than the typical three larger meals.

  - If many interventions fail but the person still entirely consumes a particular sweet food or drink then offer a second helping even if the food is a dessert. Priority should be placed on calories and maintaining self-feeding abilities rather than on providing a 'healthy diet' in advancing dementia.

- REFERRAL: For someone at risk of poor oral intake and weight loss, or if their diet is becoming limited, consult with a dietitian for nutritional assessment.

2. Only eats certain foods

- IMPORTANT NOTICE: Only eating certain foods can lead to lower intake of calories, protein, vitamins and minerals. Monitor body weight and food intake in people who prefer certain foods and refer to a dietitian if weight is lost.

- Provide cueing:

  - Describe the foods available and use a picture menu to prompt the person with other food choices. Discuss food preferences with them and/or ask family and friends for advice on preferences.

- Use life story work to discover more about the person's usual eating and drinking habits, routines and personal preferences (likes and dislikes).

- Modify table setting:

  - Try serving one food item at a time with high-calorie, high-protein foods first.

- Increase socialisation:

  - Adapting the service style may increase interest in the meal on offer, and the social interaction may stimulate eating. For example provide the opportunity for the person to serve their own food, or show the food before serving it, rather than serving pre-plated food. This can also improve portion size chosen and provide increased food choice.

  - Try eating your meal with the person. Eating with company can enhance mealtime abilities owing to social interaction and taking cues to eat from others. In addition you can help keep their focus on the meal and provide appropriate assistance if required to help maintain food intake. It can also help carers become more aware of individuals' likes, dislikes and preferences.

- Enhance familiarity:

  - Try providing simple, well-known or culturally appropriate dishes to see if this helps with recognition and consumption of other foods.

- Stimulate senses:

  - Try presenting foods in a different way, for example with or without sauces.

  - Try using additional flavours in foods, for example beef extract added to a beef dish will enhance the flavour of the beef. Remember herbs, salt and spices increase variety of flavour but do not always enhance flavour itself.

  - Trial sensory cueing involving the smell of food aromas (for example freshly baked bread, frying bacon or brewing coffe) around the mealtime. This can let the person know it is time to eat and help stimulate appetite for all foods.

- Trial foods and meals with heightened sensory input, for example salty, cold, sweet, sharp, carbonated, spicy and crunchy; or foods that make your tongue tingle, for example hot or chilli sauce, menthol and ginger. These stimulate the senses and encourage food consumption.

- Food First advice:

  - Focus on quality rather than quantity of food eaten. Trial food fortification techniques to increase calories and protein in the limited foods that are eaten, for example fortifying with additional oil (e.g. olive, sunflower) to increase calorie content. Supplementing the diet with a multivitamin tablet may also be indicated.

  - If many interventions fail but the person still entirely consumes a particular food or drink then offer a second helping even if the food is a dessert. Priority should be placed on calories and maintaining self-feeding abilities rather than on providing a 'healthy diet'.

- CARE HOME SPECIFIC: Increase socialisation:

  - Sit the person with a friend or someone they have an affinity with to enhance social interaction which may improve abilities. Or if already doing this sit them with someone who has maintained eating abilities, as this may help the person continue to feed themselves by taking cues from others.

- REFERRAL: For someone at risk of poor oral intake and weight loss, or if diet is becoming limited, consult with a dietitian for nutritional assessment.

3. Eats (or drinks) too fast

- IMPORTANT NOTICE: If the speed of eating is thought to compromise someone's safety (i.e. you witness signs of aspiration or choking) when eating or drinking, liaise with a speech and language pathologist/therapist (SLP/SLT) immediately.

- Provide cueing:
  - Use verbal cues to prompt the individual to slow down. Reassure the person that there is plenty of food available and it will not run out.

  - Manually show slower eating behaviours and techniques; for example encourage the person to completely finish each mouthful before preparing the next mouthful, or put cutlery down after each mouthful.

  - Try offering food and fluid in small portions and cut food into small pieces.

- Modify tableware:
  - Try providing smaller cutlery items so less food can be placed on the cutlery at one time.

- Increase socialisation:
  - Try eating your meal with the person. Eating with company can enhance mealtime abilities owing to social interaction and taking cues to eat from others. In addition you can help keep their focus on the meal and provide appropriate assistance if required to help maintain food intake. It can also help carers become more aware of individuals' likes, dislikes and preferences.

- Adjust environment:
  - Introduce relaxing music to suit the individual's preferences as this can improve meal behaviours. Be aware of other negative environmental influences (over- or understimulation, auditory or visual confusion, institutional appearance) and adjust as required.

- CARE HOME SPECIFIC: Consider seating arrangements:
  - Sit the person with a friend or someone they have an affinity with to enhance social interaction, which may improve abilities. Or if already doing this sit them with

someone who has maintained eating abilities as this may help the person continue to feed themselves by taking cues from others.

4. Mixes food together

- IMPORTANT NOTICE: Ignore and accept unusual ways of eating as long as the food is eaten.

- Provide cueing:

    - Check glasses are worn if normally used.

- Modify table setting:

    - Limit the visual challenges and choices by providing one plate with one type of food at a time.

- Increase socialisation:

    - Try eating your meal with the person. Eating with company can enhance mealtime abilities owing to social interaction and taking cues to eat from others. In addition you can help keep their focus on the meal and provide appropriate assistance if required to help maintain food intake. It can also help carers become more aware of individuals' likes, dislikes and preferences.

- Adjust environment:

    - Introduce relaxing music to suit someone's preferences as this can improve meal behaviours. Be aware of other negative environmental influences (over- or understimulation, auditory or visual confusion, institutional appearance) and adjust as required.

- CARE HOME SPECIFIC: Increase socialisation:

    - Consider seating arrangements. Sit the person with a friend or someone they have an affinity with to enhance social interaction, which may improve abilities. Or if already doing this sit them with someone who has maintained eating abilities as this may help the person continue to feed themselves by taking cues from others.

5. Does not eat lunch but eats breakfast and some dinner

- IMPORTANT NOTICE: Missing meals can lead to lower intake of calories, protein, vitamins and minerals. Monitor body weight and food intake in people who prefer to regularly miss meals, and refer to a dietitian if weight is lost.

- Food First advice:

  - Check that a relatively large amount of fluid or additional snacks are not being offered too close to the lunchtime as this may be impacting on someone's intake by increasing satiety.

  - Focus on quality rather than quantity of food eaten. Trial food fortification techniques to increase calories and protein, for example fortifying breakfast foods with protein powders or milk powder. Supplementing the diet with a multivitamin tablet may also be indicated.

- Modify meal pattern:

  - Trial breakfast as the main meal of the day and provide a range of different cooked breakfasts for nutritional variety. This may replace the foods not eaten at the main meal.

  - Trial changing the types of food offered at dinner time with an emphasis on more finger food choices, repeated breakfast food options and possibly more carbohydrate, which may all enhance food intake, for example boiled eggs, muffins, toast and cereal. This may replace the foods not eaten at the main meal if this meal is consistently missed.

  - Trial providing two main meals rather than three as the individual may need longer between meals to gain an appetite.

- Stimulate senses:

  - Trial sensory cueing involving the smell of food aromas (for example freshly baked bread, frying bacon or brewing coffee) around the mealtime. This can let the person know it is time to eat and help stimulate appetite for all foods.

- Increase socialisation:

    - Adapting the service style may increase interest in the meal on offer and the social interaction may stimulate eating. For example provide the opportunity for the person to serve their own food, or show the food before serving it, rather than serving pre-plated food. This can also improve portion size chosen and provide increased food choice.

    - Try eating your meal with the person. Eating with company can enhance mealtime abilities owing to social interaction and taking cues to eat from others. In addition you can help keep their focus on the meal and provide appropriate assistance if required to help maintain food intake. It can also help carers become more aware of individuals' likes, dislikes and preferences.

- Adjust environment:

    - Introduce relaxing music to suit the person's preferences as this can improve meal behaviours. Be aware of other negative environmental influences (over- or understimulation, auditory or visual confusion, institutional appearance) and adjust as required.

- Adapt food:

    - Trial finger foods at lunch to see if this increases intake. Also ensure finger food options or nourishing drinks are available to offer if the original meal is not eaten.

- Enhance familiarity:

    - Try to prepare familiar foods in familiar ways, especially foods that are favourites or culturally significant, to see if this increases intake.

- CARE HOME SPECIFIC: Consider seating arrangements:

    - Sit the person with a friend or someone they have an affinity with to enhance social interaction, which may improve abilities. Or if already doing this sit them with someone who has maintained eating abilities as this may help the person continue to feed themselves by taking cues from others.

- REFERRAL: If the person is regularly not eating lunch meals and has lost weight refer to a dietitian to assess current nutritional intake and adequacy.

6. Eats very small amounts of food (or drink)

- IMPORTANT NOTICE: Ageing can cause decreased satiety levels. However, a loss of appetite may be linked to depression or acute illness; therefore if you suspect this please first consult with a doctor.

- Provide cueing:

  - Use verbal cues and prompts, for example 'Have you nearly finished?', to encourage the individual to eat (and drink).

  - If eating with others avoid removing plates until everyone has finished as this may signal the person to stop eating.

- Modify table setting:

  - Try limiting the number of foods available at any one time. This is to prevent the person from feeling overwhelmed at the size of the meal.

- Modify meal pattern:

  - Allow the person to eat when hungry and ensure food is available at all times, rather than making them eat at set times.

  - If there is a time when the person eats more, offer extra food, second helpings, snacks or finger foods at this time.

- Modify tableware:

  - Try serving meals on a larger plate, preferably one that also contrasts in colour with the food, to make the serving size appear smaller. This may benefit those with smaller appetites and those who often do not finish their meals.

- Stimulate senses:

  - Trial sensory cueing involving the smell of food aromas (for example freshly baked bread, frying bacon or brewing coffee) around the mealtime. This can let the person know it is time to eat and help stimulate appetite for all foods.

- Increase socialisation:

  - Adapting the service style may increase interest in the meal on offer, and the social interaction may stimulate eating. For example provide the opportunity for the person to serve their own food, or show the food before serving it, rather than being served pre-plated food. This can also improve portion size chosen and provide increased food choice.

  - Try eating your meal with the person. Eating with company can enhance mealtime abilities owing to social interaction and taking cues to eat from others. In addition you can help keep their focus on the meal and provide appropriate assistance if required to help maintain food intake. It can also help carers become more aware of individuals' likes, dislikes and preferences.

- Enhance familiarity:

  - Try to prepare familiar foods in familiar ways, especially foods that are favourites or culturally significant, to see if this increases intake.

- Food First advice:

  - Try offering protein and energy (calorie) dense sources of food first so they are more likely eaten. Avoid large servings as this will deter the person from eating.

  - Focus on quality rather than quantity of food eaten. Trial food fortification techniques to increase calories and protein and ensure all small amounts of food eaten are as nutrient dense as possible. Supplementing the diet with a multivitamin tablet may also be indicated.

- Think 'little and often'. Provide regular small and nutrient-dense meals, snacks, nourishing drinks or finger foods (along with sips of fluid) throughout the day rather than the typical three larger meals.

- Trial nourishing drinks between or after meals, which may be better accepted. Often it is easier to obtain additional nutrition from liquid rather than eating more food when a small appetite is present.

- If the person is struggling to consume enough food during mealtimes then try offering protein and energy (calorie) dense sources of food first so they are more likely eaten. Avoid large servings as this may deter the individual from eating.

- Focus on quality rather than quantity of food eaten. Trial food fortification techniques to increase calories and protein and ensure all small amounts of food eaten are as nutrient dense as possible. Supplementing the diet with a multivitamin tablet may also be indicated.

- CARE HOME SPECIFIC: Increase socialisation:

  - Consider seating arrangements. Sit the person with a friend or someone they have an affinity with to enhance social interaction, which may improve abilities. Or if already doing this sit them with someone who has maintained eating abilities as this may help the person continue to feed themselves by taking cues from others.

- REFERRAL: If dietary intake is compromised and weight is lost consult with a dietitian for nutritional assessment.

7. Slow eating or prolonged mealtimes

- IMPORTANT NOTICE: If the person has dysphagia (swallowing difficulty) then a prolonged mealtime may be a risk factor for a negative health consequence (asphyxiation and/or choking episode, aspiration incidents, dehydration and poor nutritional status).

- Provide cueing:
  - Use verbal cues and prompting to encourage the person to eat throughout the meal and allow one hour or more to eat.
  - If eating with others avoid removing plates until everyone has finished as this may signal the person to stop eating.
  - At the mealtime serve small portions and replenish to help keep the food warm. If caring in the person's own home reheat food when needed. If in a care setting consult local policies for reheating of food.

- Modify tableware:
  - Trial food served on specifically designed warmed plates or plate warmers.

- Increase socialisation:
  - Adapting the service style may increase interest in the meal on offer and the social interaction may stimulate eating. For example provide the opportunity for the person to serve their own food, or show the food before serving it, rather than serving pre-plated food. This can also improve portion size chosen and provide increased food choice.
  - Try eating your meal with the person. Eating with company can enhance mealtime abilities owing to social interaction and taking cues to eat from others. In addition you can help keep their focus on the meal and provide appropriate assistance if required to help maintain food intake. It can also help carers become more aware of individuals' likes, dislikes and preferences.

- CARE HOME SPECIFIC: Consider seating arrangements. Sit the person with a friend or someone they have an affinity with to enhance social interaction, which may improve abilities. Or if already doing this sit them with someone who has maintained eating abilities as this may help the person continue to feed themselves by taking cues from others.

- Adapt food:

  - Trial finger foods as this may require less effort than using cutlery, especially if the person tires during the mealtime. Finger food can be combined with a soft diet if a texture-modified diet is recommended.

- Texture modification:

  - Trial a different food texture by providing softer foods that are easier to chew and swallow. This may be especially pertinent for those who tire during the mealtime. Use the Dysphagia Diet Food Texture Descriptors (NPSA, 2011) or IDDSI Framework and Descriptors (IDDSI, 2016) to define the correct soft consistency if a swallowing difficulty has been identified.

- Stimulate senses:

  - Trial sensory cueing involving the smell of food aromas (for example freshly baked bread, frying bacon or brewing coffee) around the mealtime. This can help stimulate appetite for foods.

- Full assistance:

  - If all suggestions fail then the person may require assistance with feeding; therefore trial full feeding assistance for two days and record and monitor food and fluid intake at mealtimes. Consider using a teaspoon to feed the person, as they may prefer small bites of food.

- REFERRAL: Consult with an occupational therapist for further assessment of specific eating needs. If dietary intake is compromised and weight is lost consult with a dietitian for nutritional assessment.

8

Oral Abilities and Behaviours

THE RELATIONSHIP WITH SWALLOWING DIFFICULTIES

Introduction

This chapter discusses the common occurrence of dysphagia (swallowing difficulties) in people living with dementia, and relates this to typical oral abilities and behaviours observed at mealtimes. Oral abilities include the ability to chew and swallow but also include related behaviours such as spitting out food or not opening the mouth. It is important to note that behavioural types of oral abilities such as refusing food or not opening the mouth can be both a sign of a swallowing difficulty but also a sign that the person's mealtime needs are not being met. This has been described as the dual diagnosis of dementia (Tristani, 2016), questioning whether it is the dementia or the swallowing difficulties triggering these symptoms.

As people with advancing dementia may not be able to communicate their needs, behaviours such as refusing to eat may arise for several different reasons. For example it may mean that they do not like the food, they are not in a supported mealtime environment or they simply do not want to eat. However, additionally this behaviour can mean that they have a swallowing difficulty, and the distinction between a behaviour and a swallowing difficulty will need to be assessed and monitored by carers. This dual diagnosis of dysphagia and dementia does not have standard guidelines to help with the management of the conditions. Instead critical thinking involving assessment and implementing interventions to preserve safety, nutrition, hydration and quality of life form the basis of care (Tristani, 2016).

The list provided below, taken from section 3 of the Dementia Mealtime Assessment Tool (DMAT), draws carers' attention to the most common oral abilities and behaviours observed at mealtimes. When oral abilities and behaviours are discussed in this chapter it is important to note that these are potentially indicators of a swallowing difficulty and as such may require investigation and treatment advice by a speech and language therapist. Highlighted in this chapter will be practical ways to manage changes in oral abilities; however when dealing with dysphagia importance must always be placed on the person's safety. If you are caring for someone who expresses the oral abilities found in the list and described in this chapter, it is critical that if any of these oral abilities are thought to compromise their safety (that is, you witness signs of choking or aspiration), then they are referred to a speech and language therapist for proper investigation as to the cause and treatment of any decreased oral abilities. It is also important that a referral is not delayed so the swallow can be accurately assessed before perhaps the dementia progresses and/or the swallow deteriorates further and then a swallow assessment is too difficult or too late to perform.

Common observed oral abilities that can affect food and fluid intake and are all potential indicators of swallowing difficulties

- Bites on cutlery (spoon, fork, knife)

- Does not open mouth

- Holds food or leaves food in mouth

- Spits out food

- Reduced ability chewing

- Prolonged chewing without swallowing

- Does not chew food before swallowing

- Reduced ability swallowing or refusing to swallow

Adapted from Durnbaugh et al. (1996); Keller et al. (2006); Crawley and Hocking (2011)

Dysphagia (swallowing difficulties)
Definition of dysphagia

Dysphagia is the medical term for swallowing difficulties; conservative estimates suggest a worldwide population prevalence of 8 per cent (Cichero *et al.*, 2013). Dysphagia is a term that covers the entire swallowing process of food and liquid from mouth to stomach. It is classified into four categories (oropharyngeal, oesophageal, oesophago-gastric and para-oesophageal) depending on where the symptom occurs. However for the purpose of this chapter, only oropharyngeal dysphagia – defined as difficulty in moving the bolus of food from the mouth to the oesophagus (throat) – will be considered, and the term swallowing difficulties will be used to describe this.

Both age-related changes to swallowing physiology (reduced saliva, thirst, muscle strength of tongue, cough reflex and increased likelihood of reflux) and primarily diseases such as dementia are predisposing risk factors for swallowing difficulties in the elderly (Sura *et al.*, 2012). Due to this the prevalence of swallowing difficulties in UK care homes can be up to 68 per cent (Patients Association, 2015) with similar prevalence rates seen in institutionalised elderly patients in Australia (40–60%) (Shanley and O'Loughlin, 2000) and in people with dementia in America (45%) (Tristani, 2016).

Symptoms to watch out for in swallowing difficulties

There are obvious signs, usually seen immediately when eating or drinking (adapted from Kellett, 2012, and Griffin *et al.*, 2009):

- coughing, choking or gagging while swallowing

- wet or gurgly voice

- throat clearing

- pocketing food in mouth

- multiple swallows on each mouthful

- perspiration on brow or watery eyes after swallow

- pain while swallowing (odynophagia)

- sensation of food stuck in throat or chest

- regurgitation, sometimes through the nose.

The less obvious signs are usually underlying symptoms of a swallowing difficulty:

- recurring chest infections/pneumonia

- unexplained weight reduction, loss of appetite, food/drink refusal

- poor control of food or saliva in the mouth (drooling)

- dehydration.

Along with a reduction in oral abilities and behaviours, if you also witness any of these signs and symptoms then a discussion with the caring team should take place, as it indicates a referral to a speech and language therapist. If you are concerned someone may be exhibiting these signs, using a checklist to record your observations to help inform a speech and language therapist can be useful. An example of a checklist of warning signs can be found on page 51 of the document 'Dining with Dementia' which is freely accessible (Griffin *et al.*, 2009). A speech and language therapist will provide guideline advice both on how to ensure safe swallowing practices specific for the person as well as good feeding techniques.

Consequences of swallowing difficulties: malnutrition and social and psychological burden

The clinical consequences of swallowing difficulties include malnutrition, dehydration, aspiration, choking, pneumonia and death (Ekberg *et al.*, 2002; Sura *et al.*, 2012; Cichero *et al.*, 2013). Swallowing difficulties can become a source of nutritional problems including decreased intake of food and/or fluid, increasing the risk of malnutrition and dehydration. A swallowing difficulty also increases the risk of choking on food or aspirating on liquid. Aspirating food or fluid is a cause of pneumonia due to the food or fluid entering the lungs and initiating infection.

The social and psychological consequences that impact on quality of life include less enjoyment of food, increased anxiety or panic at mealtimes, believing the condition is untreatable, avoiding eating with others (leading to social isolation and therefore limiting social interaction), and the feeling that having a swallowing difficulty makes life less enjoyable (Ekberg *et al.*, 2002). If you have a swallowing difficulty then eating and drinking can become an unpleasant experience and the increased anxiety experienced may be magnified in people with dementia who cannot express their concerns. Eating less due to discomfort, refusing food and drink, still feeling hungry or thirsty after a meal, lower energy and protein intakes and experiencing weight loss are all common traits associated with swallowing difficulties (Ekberg *et al.*, 2002). Elderly people living in assisted living facilities have higher rates of malnutrition if they have a swallowing difficulty compared to those who do not. Those with a swallowing difficulty tend to eat purée or fluid food more often and consume smaller food portions and less fluid (Lindroos *et al.*, 2014).

The management of swallowing difficulties

Dysphagia is under-recognised, poorly diagnosed and poorly managed therefore referral to the appropriate professionals at the right time is paramount to the person's health and safety. In a pan-European study of people living with dysphagia and serious medical conditions including dementia, only 40 per cent of those surveyed had received a confirmed diagnosis of dysphagia while only 32 per cent received treatment by healthcare professionals (Ekberg *et al.*, 2002). Interestingly participants from the UK were more likely to receive a diagnosis than other European countries but once they received this diagnosis were less likely to be treated. UK participants were also less likely to inform healthcare professionals or even relatives of their difficulties, which may be one factor for a lack of treatment. Access to speech and language therapists through the NHS may be another reason for lack of treatment especially for those living in care homes where access will be different in various parts of the UK. A survey by the Patients Association found different experiences from getting access to speech and language therapist after care staff had identified a swallowing difficulty, with some experiencing a prompt service but others experiencing delays (the Patients Association, 2015). If the person living with dementia and dysphagia does not or cannot complain about their swallowing difficulties, and care staff are unaware of the signs of dysphagia or risk factors associated with swallowing difficulties at mealtimes, then clearly no interventions to manage swallowing difficulties will be implemented. It is the opinion of many authors and patient charities (Ekberg *et al.*, 2002; Lindroos *et al.*, 2014; the Patients Association, 2015) that training for care staff on awareness of swallowing difficulties, and correct management by speech and language therapists or appropriate qualified healthcare personnel, should be the gold-standard approach to managing people with dementia who have this condition.

Unfortunately this is not always possible. Improved recognition of swallowing difficulties and their management can help improve quality of life and hopefully prevent adverse events such as choking episodes and death. Any such adverse events or other symptoms witnessed by carers at mealtimes, or when observing any of the oral abilities and behaviours highlighted in section 3 of the Dementia Mealtime Assessment Tool, should act as a prompt to care staff to seek professional expert help. The identification of reduced oral abilities and behaviours and the implementation of interventions should also not be used as a replacement for speech and language input if this is indicated.

Swallowing difficulties and oral abilities in dementia

Swallowing difficulties are a common symptom of dementia leading to changes in texture of food and liquid consumed (Sura *et al.*, 2012). The prevalence of swallowing difficulties in people with dementia ranges from 13 per cent to 57 per cent (Alagiakrishnan, Bhanji and Kurian, 2013). In those with later-stage dementia roughly 50 per cent to 90 per cent experience swallowing difficulties and a reduction in oral abilities with mortality seen in 39 per cent of these at six months (Chan and Kwan, 2014). For those with dementia living in long-term care, estimates suggest up to 45 per cent can experience some degree of swallowing difficulties (Sura *et al.*, 2012). A seminal study on all mealtime abilities found that out of 349 older adults living in care homes 68 per cent exhibited signs of dysphagia (Steele *et al.*, 1997). Higher prevalence rates of swallowing difficulties are seen in those with advanced dementia and increased cognitive decline (Lindroos *et al.*, 2014). It has been estimated that people with dementia will spend about 40 per cent of their years living with the condition in the severe stage (Tristani, 2016). Carers are therefore likely to witness a decline in oral abilities and at some point in the advancing dementia there is higher probability that the person will experience swallowing difficulties. The reduction in common oral abilities listed above is also commonly seen with other reduced mealtime abilities including the ability to feed oneself as discussed in Chapter 4 (Sura *et al.*, 2012). This means the person with dementia has increased dependence on carers to provide their nutritional requirements in a safe and nutritious form.

Swallowing difficulties and oral behaviours in dementia

The different oral abilities and behaviours commonly observed at mealtimes in people with dementia and shown in the list above can all be considered as potential indicators of swallowing difficulties. Apart from indicating potential swallowing difficulties they can also indicate behaviours as a sign of an unmet need. Behaviours at mealtimes and the belief that they relate to an unmet need or indicate the person is not being fully supported were discussed in Chapter 2. In the list above several reduced oral abilities could also be observed as behaviours; for example, 'Does not open mouth' or 'Refusing to swallow' could be perceived as a refusal to eat rather than a sign that a swallowing difficulty is present. Similarly 'Spits out food' could indicate a refusal to eat rather than a sign of swallowing difficulties, or quite simply it could be that the person does not like the food or that it is too hot/cold and so on. The person with dementia communicates this by spitting out the food. It can be difficult to distinguish oral abilities between a behaviour and a swallowing difficulty. This is why if any signs of aspiration or choking or other adverse events are observed a referral to a speech and language therapist is a priority to ensure correct management.

Specific effective interventions for the management of swallowing difficulties or a reduction in oral abilities and behaviours in those with dementia are limited and unclear (Alagiakrishnan *et al.*, 2013).

The evidence for managing oral abilities, behaviours and swallowing difficulties

Speyer *et al.*'s (2010) review of speech and language therapy notes that the effectiveness of interventions used in the management of swallowing difficulties is unclear; however, most have a positive impact on outcomes. Nonetheless they also note that due to a lack of strong evidence, conclusions from studies cannot be generalised or compared, therefore making it challenging to determine which intervention is likely to be the most effective. As swallowing difficulties present such a huge risk to the person the management of oral abilities is centred on patient safety and consists of two main interventions. The first is texture-modified foods, for example soft or puréed, and the second is thickened fluids; both are described in this chapter. To maintain the safe oral intake of food and fluids it has been said that providing the modified food and fluid is a necessity rather than a choice for the person with swallowing difficulties (Cichero *et al.*, 2013). Research into dysphagia and people with dementia is fraught with difficulties, especially considering it would be unethical to randomise people into a group not receiving an intervention where one of the outcomes of this approach could be an increased choking risk and death (Cichero *et al.*, 2013).

The evidence for effective management of a reduction in oral abilities and behaviours associated with dementia when a swallowing difficulty is not indicated is also not conclusive and requires further exploration. There are several caring techniques, enhancing familiarity of foods and modifications to the sensory input of foods that can be of benefit and will be discussed.

This chapter will try to draw out the practical application of interventions for enhancing oral abilities and behaviours from research and other literature. Importantly the reader should bear in mind that just because an intervention is recommended to be trialled to support someone it does not mean it will be successful. Determining the effectiveness of an intervention in terms of safety, increased nutrition and hydration or preserving quality of life involves clinical reasoning and should be accounted for when assessing effectiveness. It is likely that several interventions will need to be trialled and monitored to find the most appropriate and effective one. There is one final thought you should also keep in mind. When managing oral abilities there is the risk of swallowing difficulties being present; therefore the person's safety should be at the forefront of any intervention.

All the evidence discussed in this section is related to the practical interventions provided in the next chapter.

Cueing

As discussed in Chapter 4, providing cueing in the form of verbal and manual prompts can be a simple and effective caring technique while increasing engagement with the person with dementia. Some commonly used cueing techniques to prompt someone to chew or swallow their food are provided in the interventions section in the subsequent practical solutions chapter. For example if someone has 'Prolonged chewing without swallowing' then providing cueing by manually prompting the individual by presenting an empty spoon or fork back up towards the mouth, as if you are offering the next mouthful, may remind them to swallow (Griffin et al., 2009). Or if someone has a 'Reduced ability swallowing or refusing to swallow' then softly stroking their arm or using calming rhythmic patting and talking to them about the food can help swallowing if refusal is seen. The effectiveness of these interventions has not been fully evaluated in those with reduced oral abilities but they do provide useful non-invasive caring techniques that can be successful.

Posture

Someone's posture at mealtimes, although not strictly related to cueing, is still a very important part of management. The correct postural position at a mealtime can help reduce the risk of aspiration and make it easier for the person to eat and drink, therefore helping to reduce fatigue at the mealtime related to swallowing difficulty (Griffin et al., 2009). It is imperative that a speech and language therapist is consulted to help achieve the most appropriate postural positions for eating and drinking in those who have a diagnosed swallowing difficulty, to ensure a safe and effective swallow.

Oral health

Oral and dental health can be ignored in individuals with later-stage dementia but it may be another factor affecting nutritional intake and changes in taste that can lead to a reduction in oral abilities and behaviours. For those living in care homes, as dementia advances it can have a deleterious effect on oral health (Adam and Preston, 2006). Despite there being no published studies on the management of dental health issues in people with dementia there are treatment planning publications, and clearly maintaining oral health is extremely important (BDA, 2013). Having said this, research is always evolving, and there is one ongoing study investigating the effect of increasing masticatory activity (achieved by three different actions: providing oral health care, increasing food consistency, or a combination of both) and evaluating if this has a positive effect on quality of life (including cognition, mood and activities of daily living) of older people with dementia (Weijenberg et al., 2013).

From a nutrition perspective oral health issues can affect the ability to eat and may unnecessarily trigger a change in the texture of food consumed. Poor oral health can also impact on self-esteem, dignity and social interaction, therefore affecting both health and wellbeing (Alzheimer's Society, 2016). The checking and monitoring of oral health should be a regular part of care for people with dementia as it is for anyone else. If the oral abilities listed in the introduction to the chapter are observed at mealtimes then a check of any oral health issues should be considered and ruled out as a possible cause of change in oral abilities. Most care homes or NHS organisations will likely have a protocol for assessing oral health. The National Institute for Health and Care Excellence (NICE) has developed guidelines for oral health for adults in care homes; in the resources section is an oral health assessment tool which is freely and easily accessible to anyone (NICE, 2016). For more dementia-specific guidance other freely available resources are on the internet and the reader is referred to these (Halton Region Health Department, 2012) and advised to obtain training from an appropriate experienced professional. If potential issues are discovered then an assessment by a dentist would be indicated, or for general oral health practices an oral health professional, dentist or dental hygienist may be needed to provide specific advice for individuals. Certainly if swallowing difficulties as well as oral health issues have been identified then specific management for both of these conditions becomes more complex. If someone uses dentures it is worth noting that these can slow the rate of chewing, and poorly fitting dentures may contribute or aggravate oral abilities (Steele et al., 1997).

Oral behaviours

Until appropriate assessment has been instigated it is often not known if a refusal to open the mouth when food or drink is presented is due to a swallowing difficulty or indicates oral apraxia (Tristani, 2016). Limited research has looked at ways to manage this. One study however conducted by speech and language therapists in Hong Kong described their observations and interventions for supporting individuals (Chan and Kwan, 2014). The authors drew from previous research to describe oral abilities falling into four categories:

1. swallowing difficulties with risk of aspiration

2. refusal of food by verbal or physical rejection and oral defensiveness (relates to 'Does not open mouth' or 'Refusing to swallow')

3. oral spitting and spillage (relates to 'Spits out food')

4. food retention (relates to 'Holds food or leaves food in the mouth').

This study was conducted in Hong Kong, where often the emphasis of care is on 'feeding' the person with dementia, and as such some of the successful interventions they adopted would not be recognised as suitable in the UK for older adults with dementia. In fact they are more often seen used in paediatrics, for example using bottle feeding or teat soothing to minimise oro-motor reflexes. Many interventions they did use, however, certainly would be used in the UK: the results from the study indicated the following:

1. To reduce refusal they used 'behaviour modification' by rhythmical patting, music and conditioning with favourite foods in the diet.

2. To initiate oral anticipation they used oral stimulation by alternation of food appetisers with specific taste and temperature.

3. To enhance recognition of eating using 'cognitive psychological adaptation' they used a selected specific carer to provide feeding and provide a recognised voice and verbal prompting.

As mentioned 'feeding' is the main emphasis of treatment and in fact the continued ability to 'feed' the people with dementia in the intervention group was the main outcome, with the participants in the study having many reduced mealtime abilities. The researchers found that using the interventions led to improved feeding even at six months follow-up and also led to a reduction of readmissions to the speech and language therapy team.

In summary this interesting study showed that supporting physical refusal and oral abilities using music and calming rhythmic patting can be effective. To support verbal refusal using favourite foods and selected carers with recognised faces and voices can also be effective. Although not included in this study, the use of family members who should have recognisable voices and faces would be another intervention option to support verbal refusal of foods. For a mixture of behaviours then a mix of all interventions can be tried. These associations between refusing food and effectiveness of the interventions in reducing food refusal need to be further substantiated; and to see if they improve outcomes such as food intake, weight gain and quality of life, however, they provide further ideas to manage this difficult subject. The authors also mention how a dedicated and devoted team (as used in their research) is needed to produce effective outcomes, something which is not always reproducible in normal care settings.

Sensory adaptation

The importance of the senses for food intake and enjoyment was discussed in Chapter 6; additional sensory stimulation can also be used to enhance oral abilities. For example to help stimulate chewing and swallowing, a range of foods with heightened sensory properties can be trialled and have been used to some effect (Chan and Kwan, 2014; Tristani, 2016). Cold or alternating temperatures and sharp, sour, sweet, carbonated, salty, spicy foods and drinks can be used as food appetisers or within meals to provide the sensory stimulation.

Adapted food
Soft diet
It can be common for someone living with dementia to have a soft diet despite not having any swallowing difficulties. General weakness,

not feeling well, poor dentition or even just that it is easier for them to eat mean a soft diet can be a simple and effective choice. If someone is consuming a soft diet but has no swallowing difficulty they do not need a texture-modified soft diet (see the next section).

It is important to consider that even if someone does not clearly show signs of a swallowing difficulty, if they require soft foods they may be at risk of swallowing difficulties. The reduction in 'bite force' is significantly reduced in people with swallowing difficulties and is also related to the number of teeth affecting the ability to chew. Deterioration in health and weakened muscles associated with the function of ageing also impact the ability to chew with effective force. The use of dentures is common in elderly people and this may also present a higher risk factor for swallowing difficulties due to the loss of specific sensations associated with the perception of the force and pressure required to chew. For example the sensation of crisp or crunchy food can be reduced in those with dentures and fewer teeth (Cichero et al., 2013). Therefore for those who require soft food or for their food to be cut into small bites, or who use dentures, then increased awareness of swallowing difficulties must be maintained.

Purée diet

Similarly to a soft diet for some people with dementia, acceptance of a purée diet may be indicated despite not having a swallowing difficulty. As dementia advances it is not uncommon for the texture of the food to change from a normal diet to a completely liquid diet as shown in Figure 8.1. Adapting the consistency of food becomes an important intervention to maintain sufficient food intake, nutrition and hydration. If the purée diet is required for someone with swallowing difficulties then compliance with safety guidelines to avoid the risk of choking and aspiration is indicated; this is discussed later in this chapter. Whether this is indicated or not, ensuring the food looks appealing and contains appropriate nutritional content should be the focus. Information on these important aspects is a book in itself; further information can be obtained from charitable resources including the Caroline Walker Trust (Crawley and Hocking, 2011) and Hammond Care in association with Maggie Beer and the Dementia Centre (Hammond Care, 2014).

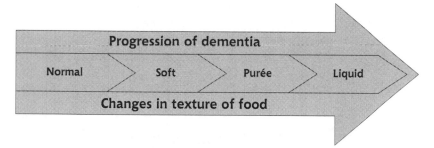

Figure 8.1: *Changes in texture of food as dementia progresses*

Liquid diets

In the later stages of dementia foods of a more drinkable nature may be indicated; therefore providing high-calorie soups, hot cereals (protein breakfast shakes), milkshakes and other nourishing drinks may be more appropriate than food. This is especially useful if the person with dementia has maintained more abilities to drink than to eat and they continue to feed themselves via a drinking cup. A dietitian should be consulted to check nutritional adequacy, and ensuring presentation of a liquid diet in attractive tableware should be given extra effort.

Texture-Modified Diets (TMDs)

Texture-modified diets (TMDs) are foods that have been adapted to a consistency that is safe for consumption by people with diagnosed dysphagia (swallowing difficulties). You may see or read dysphagia or swallowing difficulties described as an 'unsafe swallow'. This does not mean it is unsafe for the person to eat or drink and that they should stop but rather the appropriate food texture is required and used. It is critical that an expert in dysphagia makes decisions and provides clear guidance on what TMDs are used for each individual. This guidance should be provided to all care staff as confusion over food textures has contributed to death in some cases (Cichero *et al.*, 2013). In the UK currently (2017) it is recommended to use the National Patient Safety Agency (2011) Dysphagia Diet Food Texture Descriptors (NPSA, 2011) to determine the correct texture modification. This UK-based set of guidelines provides standard terminology for describing the correct consistency of foods suitable for the safety of people with dysphagia.

Estimates suggest between 15 and 30 per cent of food is modified in texture in long-term care facilities (Cichero *et al.*, 2013) indicating a huge demand and need for appropriate TMDs and the catering skills required for this. In a seminal study on mealtime abilities in 349 older adults living in long-term care 68 per cent of them had dysphagia and 48 per cent (159 out of 349) received a texture-modified diet (Steele *et al.*, 1997). For those providing TMDs in health and care settings the UK guidelines recommend that nationally recognised terminology is used to describe the consistency of four food textures as shown in Table 8.1.

Table 8.1: Dysphagia diet texture descriptors for texture-modified diets

'Normal food'		< TMDs >		'Purée'	
Regular	E = Fork mashable dysphagia diet	D = Pre-mashed dysphagia diet	C = Thick purée dysphagia diet	B = Thin purée dysphagia diet

Adapted from NPSA (2011); Cichero *et al.* (2013)

Textures C and E are recommended to be available in all care settings with the other textures, or variations of them, depending on a speech and language therapist's (SLT) assessment and recommendations for individuals. This is an important document to be aware of whether you are a caterer, healthcare professional or carer.

Even though the Dysphagia Diet Food Texture Descriptors are a fantastic resource and certainly useful from a safety point of view, it must be highlighted that the guidelines do not cover the nutritional adequacy of TMDs (or thickened fluids) and neither do they address the acceptability of these modified foods and fluids with the person with dementia. Also the descriptors are not based on research evidence as unfortunately there is no strong evidence base for TMD although they are best-practice guidelines. Additionally there have been no studies comparing the benefit or effectiveness of using these guidelines compared to a standardised approach of modifying food (Sura *et al.*, 2012). Despite these limitations it is highly recommended to use the Dysphagia Diet Food Texture Descriptors by several professional organisations and this book strongly advises this too.

The main purpose of TMDs is to provide food which is safe to consume without increasing the risk of choking or asphyxiation. This is an important point to consider as safety is placed ahead of nutritional adequacy and acceptability of the modified food and fluid

(Sura *et al.*, 2012). In UK hospitals older people consuming texture-modified diets can have lower intakes of energy (calories) and protein compared to normal diets, and purée foods can contain a lower nutritional content (Wright *et al.*, 2005). Similarly in care home settings older people consuming TMD had lower intakes of calories, protein, fluid and fibre (Bannerman and McDermott, 2011). As there are no regulations in place to ensure TMDs meet nutritional standards it may be necessary for the catering team to work with a dietitian to check nutritional suitability of the TMD recipes. Modifying the texture of food and fluid is complex and can often lead to the food looking rather unappealing both in terms of taste and appearance. This in turn can lead to less food being consumed and increase the risks of malnutrition which tend to be higher in those with dysphagia. Individuals placed on a TMD can show poor adherence so it is important their actual intake is monitored. Using moulds to shape the texture-modified food will make it look much more appealing and can increase intake (Farrer *et al.*, 2015). Importantly TMDs may result in decreased food and nutrition intake with some evidence suggesting that if not used correctly TMDs can lead to over-restricted diets (Sura *et al.*, 2012); therefore having guidelines available may safeguard against this. A key practical point to take from one study that compared a standard TMD with a TMD with expanded meal options found significantly greater intake in the latter group (Sura *et al.*, 2012). Having a choice of TMD meals and not just a limited repeated range can therefore improve food intake and weight gain.

Finally it is also worth remembering that those on a TMD also tend to have more advanced dementia, ill health, decreased appetite and reduced mealtime abilities, which all impact on food and fluid intake (Lee and Song, 2015).

Thickened fluids and puréed foods

The risk of aspiration and chest infections is a concern for people with swallowing difficulties as these can both threaten life. The safety of the swallow of liquids is formally evaluated by a speech and language therapist, and once assessed an intervention involving the thickening of fluids or puréed foods may be appropriate. This thickening is done by adding different measures of powdered starch-based or gum-based thickening agents to fluids to thicken them to different levels. There are also some foods and ingredients which can be used to thicken foods such as cornflour, arrowroot, mashed potato, gravy and custard powder (Premier Foods, 2014), although perhaps a more advanced skill level is required to obtain the desired thickness as outlined below when using these ingredients. Currently in the UK (2018) the different thickness levels or 'stages' of fluids are described in Table 8.2.

Table 8.2: Different stages of thickened fluids for dysphagia diets

'Water-like'		< Fluid consistency >		'Pudding thick'
Thin	Naturally thick	Thickened fluid – stage 1 For example nectar	Thickened fluid – stage 2 For example honey	Thickened fluid – stage 3 For example pudding

Adapted from Cichero *et al.* (2013)

The research evidence on the clinical effectiveness of the different stages of thickened fluids in the management of fluid-swallowing difficulties is limited (Sura *et al.*, 2012; Cichero *et al.*, 2013); nonetheless it is the cornerstone in managing swallowing difficulties. In dementia specifically the use of thickened fluids as an evidence-based practice cannot be concluded however thickened fluids may be effective if set guidelines are adhered to. The acceptability of thickened fluids for people with dementia and dysphagia is often not reported but they have been found to be acceptable (Hines *et al.*, 2010). There is a perception that if the fluid is thick it will be safer to swallow; but one of the few randomised controlled trials in people with dementia has shown this not to be the case with a higher incidence of pneumonia in those receiving stage-3 compared to stage-1 fluid thickness (Cichero *et al.*, 2013). This highlights the importance of obtaining professional help in determining the correct consistency of thickened fluid. It is not as simple as increasing the thickness of fluid; indeed there are practical difficulties related to ensuring the correct thickness of fluid when using thickening agents. For example one study demonstrated how fluids thickened by clinicians were significantly different to those prepared in the laboratory yet the same instructions were used in both circumstances (Cichero *et al.*, 2013). To overcome these practical difficulties training on the use of thickening agents, preferably by a speech and language therapist, would be the gold standard. This is not always possible in UK care settings. If SLTs working for the NHS are unable to provide this service then it's often necessary to buy in training packages for care homes that receive little help with the practical aspects of this type of care. Alternatively pre-thickened fluids are available to purchase although the cost of this compared to setting the fluid thickness yourself is increased; it does provide consistency however.

Another concern from the use of thickened fluids is the increased risk of dehydration. Compliance with thickened fluids is often reduced, leading to less fluid being consumed (Sura *et al.*, 2012). Changes to the texture and flavour of thickened drinks may partly account for decreased intake. Experts on the topic encourage clinicians to prescribe the minimal level of thickness needed for swallowing safety to ensure hydration is maintained (Cichero, 2013). The reasons for this include feelings of satiety and thirst growing with increasingly viscous fluids, and that flavour can deteriorate with increasing thickness, both contributing to dehydration.

As shown above, although there are guidelines on creating appropriate thickness of fluids individual judgement will need to be made for different fluids. This becomes a trial-and-error approach at first: some fluids will hold their thickness consistency longer than others while some may continue to thicken. Practically this means different fluids will require different amounts of thickener to provide the same consistency. Following the manufacturers' instructions is recommended and for many their websites provide useful guidance. Unfortunately however the different thickeners can have different instructions on how to thicken so do not assume all thickeners are the same. Practical tips for carers on this topic can be found in an excellent blog post by dementia advocate Beth Britton (Britton, 2012), from chef Preston Walker (Premier Foods, 2014) and in an article by a dietitian who consumed both thickened fluids and a texture-modified C diet to gain practical knowledge (Taylor, 2016). Whenever thickening foods and fluids always check against guidelines to ensure you have achieved the correct consistency (NPSA, 2011; IDDSI, 2016).

Key practical tips for carers and people with dementia

- Make sure all carers and people with dementia are aware there is a range of thickening powders available, all of which have a slightly different taste. Therefore a change in thickening powder may help with acceptance of thickened fluid.

- Allow 'standing' time for rehydration of thickening powders as it can take several minutes for the powder to fully thicken the fluid.

- Lumps of thickener can prevent consumption of the drink. If you feel this is a problem for the person with dementia use a blender for a few seconds to create a smooth consistency before serving.

- Foods with a high water content (e.g. naturally thick soup, yoghurt, puréed fruit) may be better accepted than drinks that are thickened. As Taylor (2016) put it: 'You expect certain foods to be thick and creamy; you don't expect your tea or water to be like this.'

- Milk and fortified milk can be difficult to thicken without making the milk feel curdled, affecting its palatability. Blending the milk with fruit into a smoothie and then thickening may help overcome this problem.

- Gum-based thickeners contain fibre which throughout a day of drinking thickened fluids and/or meals can amount to a lot of additional fibre (4 to 18g/day). Increases in fibre can trigger gastro-intestinal symptoms such as bloating, pain, flatulence, diarrhoea and constipation; therefore monitoring those who cannot express changes in these symptoms would be advisable to prevent discomfort.

Adapted from Taylor (2016) and Premier Foods (2014)

There are more pre-thickened drinks becoming available so there is no need to use thickening powders but these usually work out more expensive. These include prescribed oral nutrition supplements. Both of these may be particularly useful when carers lack experience of swallowing difficulties and/or making thickened fluids. It is the opinion of the European Society for Swallowing Disorders that new thickening agents should be developed that do not have such negative effects on residue, palatability and treatment compliance caused by increasing the viscosity of fluid. Their White Paper also concludes that there is sufficient evidence for thickening fluids reducing the risk of aspiration (Newman *et al.*, 2016).

International Dysphagia Diet Standardisation Initiative

At the time of this book going to press an announcement by NHS England and a range of stakeholders has indicated that the UK will adopt an international set of standards for dysphagia diets known as the International Dysphagia Diet Standardisation Initiative (IDDSI) Framework (IDDSI, 2016) as shown in Figure 8.2. The IDDSI includes both food and fluid guidelines which are slightly different to the UK-based guidelines. The Dysphagia Diet Food Texture Descriptors (NPSA, 2011) are currently (2018) recommended for use in the UK, and the standard use of these in health care will help provide consistency in the types of textures of food suitable for people with dysphagia. Once the IDDSI framework is adopted a new set of guidelines will need to be implemented but clearly a transition process will need to be adopted. The IDDSI estimate that all food manufacturers and healthcare settings are fully IDDSI compliant by April 2019. The current Dysphagia Diet Food Texture Descriptors are not unsafe and certainly should be adhered to. One reason for adopting the new IDDSI framework is that it includes the same framework being used across different countries – meaning a common international terminology for describing TMDs – which should make both patient safety and research of effectiveness of the IDDSI on health outcomes improved and more robust. Additionally and most practically the IDDSI can combine within one framework the descriptors for both texture-modified food and fluids. Fluids and the thickening of these to make them safe for those with dysphagia are not currently addressed by the UK Dysphagia Diet Food Texture Descriptors so this is a very welcome improvement from this new framework. For additional information and to stay up to date on further implementation of the IDDSI framework visit the IDDSI website.[1]

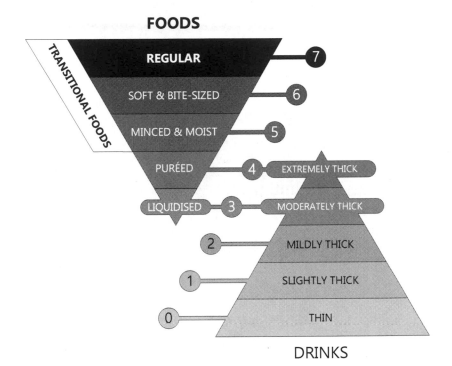

Figure 8.2: *The International Dysphagia Diet Standardisation Initiative (IDDSI) Framework 2016*
©The International Dysphagia Diet Standardisation Initiative 2016 @ http://iddsi.org/framework

Further interventions

Increased assistance needs for those with swallowing difficulties is common. Self-managing swallowing difficulties leads people to eat and swallow more slowly, taking sips of fluid between bites of food, chewing food for longer before swallowing and using special utensils (Ekberg *et al.*, 2002). Indeed the use of specially adapted utensils (which are recommended as potential interventions in

---

1   www.iddsi.org

the next practical solutions chapter to support swallowing difficulties) may also help improve outcomes (Sura *et al.*, 2012) although no strong evidence base exits.

For those who require feeding from a carer evidence points to targeted 'feeding training' of carers, which can result in increased energy and protein intakes in elderly hospital patients. Potentially a lack of training for care staff on feeding someone with a swallowing difficulty could increase the risk of an adverse event such as aspiration owing to factors such as rapid and uncontrolled presentation of food (Sura *et al.*, 2012).

Postural changes to the body and/or head along with swallow manoeuvres intended to improve the safety and efficiency of the swallow may also be recommended by speech and language therapists in addition to modification of food and fluid (Sura *et al.*, 2012).

Finally the environment at the mealtime, as discussed in detail in Chapter 10, may have an important part to play in helping to improve the safety, monitoring and intake of food and fluid. By providing a mealtime free of distractions care staff can focus on individual needs, especially of those with swallowing difficulties.

The next chapter combines the evidence discussed here into practical interventions that can be targeted at the identified reduced oral abilities and behaviours to improve the support provided.

9

Practical Interventions Section 3

MANAGING ORAL ABILITIES AND BEHAVIOURS

Assessment

Table 9.1 shows section 3 of the Dementia Mealtime Assessment Tool (DMAT, 2017) as described in Chapter 3. This section focuses on assessing oral abilities and behaviours often observed in people with later-stage dementia. Use the table for assessment of mealtime oral abilities. Regular assessment may be required, for example every month or more frequently such as weekly if you have concerns about a particular person. The interventions following the assessment are recommended for enhancing and supporting the oral abilities and behaviours of the person with dementia.

Table 9.1: The DMAT section 3: Assessment of oral abilities and behaviours

Mealtime observations: Oral abilities and behaviours	Please tick observed abilities		
	Not seen	Seen once	Seen repeatedly
1. Bites on cutlery (spoon, fork, knife)			
2. Does not open mouth			
3. Holds food or leaves food in mouth			
4. Spits out food			
5. Reduced ability chewing			
6. Prolonged chewing without swallowing			
7. Does not chew food before swallowing			
8. Reduced ability swallowing or refusing to swallow			

Carer awareness and assessment of risk factors for swallowing difficulties are important in obtaining expert help and managing a reduction of adverse events. An awareness of common oral abilities and behaviours as indicated in the DMAT may help inform carers to make better-informed treatment options and referrals to appropriate professionals.

Interventions
Guidance for interventions

- As described previously the interventions follow a hierarchy of suggestions starting with simple cueing techniques and checking oral health, then moving on to discovering personal preferences, stimulation or recognition of foods, texture modification, behaviour modification and referral to appropriate healthcare professionals.

- Training for dysphagia awareness and management (including feeding techniques, appropriate referral to speech and language therapists and providing TMDs and thickened fluids) is important. Healthcare catering teams have a huge responsibility to provide a variety of texture-modified diets (TMDs) including main meals and snacks. If care staff have not received adequate training this should be a priority for the care organisation.

- Try one or two interventions per ability at a time and monitor effectiveness. Many interventions will overlap with each other and some interventions have not been shown to be more effective than others so a multicomponent intervention approach is best used.

- There is also a need for carers to be aware of both the cognitive reasons (e.g. environmental interactions and other mealtime abilities) and the physical reasons (swallowing difficulties) for the oral abilities and behaviours observed.

- IMPORTANT NOTICE: Be aware that for any identified oral abilities and behaviours there may be risk of a swallowing difficulty being present which can impact the person's safety.

Each intervention section related to an observed oral ability or behaviour will highlight an 'IMPORTANT NOTICE' to the carer to prompt this awareness. If the safety of the person is thought to be compromised by their ability to swallow then a referral to a speech and language therapist may be indicated before any interventions are to be put in place.

Suggested interventions for supporting oral abilities and behaviours at mealtimes

1. Bites on cutlery (spoon, fork, knife)

- IMPORTANT NOTICE: People with dementia may be very sensitive to having cutlery in the mouth, for example a cold metal spoon. Avoid hard metal cutlery, large cutlery or easily breakable utensils. Lightweight but durable plastic cutlery is recommended, such as specialist polycarbonate cutlery.

- Check oral health:
    - Check for inadequate or missing dentition, loose dentures, sores, ulcers or broken teeth.

- Provide cueing:
    - Place food or utensils in the person's hand and trial using hand-under-hand technique to initiate and guide self-feeding. Also offer encouragement.

- Adapt food:
    - Trial finger foods if the problem persists and is affecting food intake. Finger food can be combined with a soft diet if a TMD is recommended.

    - After exhausting all appropriate treatment interventions (including referral), trial a cup rather than using a spoon if a purée or liquid meal is appropriate for the person, and encourage self-feeding.

- REFERRAL: If the biting on cutlery persists liaise with a speech and language pathologist /therapist (SLP/SLT) and occupational therapist (OT) for further advice.

2. Does not open mouth

- IMPORTANT NOTICE: Do not attempt to force-feed. Following several attempts to prompt the person to eat, if they still do not open their mouth then stop the meal to prevent distressing them.

- Provide cueing:

  - Offer verbal cues and verbal prompting to encourage the person to open their mouth.

  - Manually and visually show how to open mouth by 'modelling' the task a few times so the person can copy your movements.

  - Manually prompt the person by touching their lips with a spoon to initiate opening mouth.

  - Softly stroking the person's arm or using calming rhythmic patting and talking to them about the food can help encourage opening the mouth and eating.

- Sensory adaptation:

  - Trial food with a strong aroma when eating or similar smells to act as stimulation before and during the mealtime.

  - Trial food appetisers with heightened sensory input, for example salty, cold, sweet, sharp, carbonated, spicy or crunchy. Alternate between different foods to encourage the person to start eating. Use the Dysphagia Diet Food Texture Descriptors or IDDSI Framework and Descriptors to define the correct food consistency if a swallowing difficulty has been identified.

- Enhance familiarity:

  - Present favourite foods to initiate opening of the mouth and eating then offer the original meal or further foods.

  - The person may benefit from receiving assistance or recognising the voice from one specific carer, or have consistency in caring (and feeding) practices. With advancing dementia people need to recognise their carers or somehow realise they are there to assist with eating.

- Ask if a family member can help to encourage the person to eat.

- Adapt food:

  - Prepare and present food in an appetising way. For example serve puréed foods separately in moulds (not all mixed together) to help preserve individual flavours and colours.

  - Trial finger foods if the problem persists and is affecting food intake. Finger food can be combined with a soft diet if a TMD is recommended.

  - After exhausting all appropriate treatment interventions (including referral), trial a cup rather than using a spoon if a purée or liquid meal is appropriate, and encourage self-feeding.

- Adjust environment:

  - Introduce relaxing music to suit the person's preferences. Negative environmental influences at mealtimes include visual overstimulation in a crowded room and auditory confusion secondary to background noise. Adjusting one or more of these negative environmental influences may improve behaviour.

- REFERRAL: If the refusal to open mouth persists liaise with a speech and language pathologist/therapist (SLP/SLT) for further advice.

3. Holds food or leaves food in mouth

- IMPORTANT NOTICE: Holding food in the mouth can indicate a swallowing difficulty. If choking is a hazard or holding/leaving food in the mouth is thought to compromise someone's safety (i.e. you witness signs of aspiration) when eating or drinking liaise with a speech and language pathologist/therapist (SLP/SLT) immediately.

- Check oral health:

  - Check for inadequate or missing dentition, loose dentures or sores, ulcers and broken teeth.

- Provide cueing:

  - Use verbal prompts and manual cues to clear the remaining food using their tongue.

  - Manually prompt the person to swallow by massaging the jaw and cheek gently to encourage movement of food.

  - Manually prompt the person to swallow by stroking the throat gently, which can encourage swallowing.

  - Use a coated or empty spoon or spoon with a tiny bit of liquid/food to stimulate the action of chewing and/or swallowing.

- Sensory adaptation:

  - Trial food appetisers with heightened sensory input, for example salty, cold, sweet, sharp, carbonated, spicy or crunchy. Alternate between different foods to encourage the person to start eating. Use the Dysphagia Diet Food Texture Descriptors or IDDSI Framework and Descriptors to define the correct food consistency if a swallowing difficulty has been identified.

  - Offering teaspoons or sips of ice-cold drinks before and during a meal will stimulate stronger swallows and help to clear remaining oral residue (thickened fluids may be required if a swallowing difficulty has been identified). Use the Dysphagia Diet Food Texture Descriptors or IDDSI Framework and Descriptors to define the correct consistency.

  - Try alternating temperature and taste within meals, for example, warm stewed apple with ice-cream, or curry with yoghurt.

- Texture modification:

  - Trial a different food texture by providing softer foods that are easier to chew and swallow. Use the Dysphagia Diet Food Texture Descriptors or IDDSI Framework and Descriptors to define the correct soft consistency if a swallowing difficulty has been identified.

- REFERRAL: If the holding or leaving food in mouth persists, liaise with an SLP/SLT for further advice.

4. Spits out food

- IMPORTANT NOTICE: If the spitting out of food is thought to compromise the safety of the person (i.e. you witness signs of aspiration) when eating or drinking liaise with a speech and language pathologist/therapist (SLP/SLT) immediately.

- Individual references:

  - Reassess if this food is still liked; if a person with dementia does not like a food they may spit it out. Make sure food preferences (including cultural and religious) are recorded and ask family or friends for information on food habits and preferences.

  - Monitor and keep a record of types of food spat out to establish if there is a pattern (for example preferring sweet food, disliking salty food; temperature of food, seasoning).

  - Monitor if the person spits out and seems to dislike certain food textures, for example mixed food consistencies or lumps in food. If this is the case adapt the food appropriately. Use the Dysphagia Diet Food Texture Descriptors or IDDSI Framework and Descriptors to define the correct food consistency if a swallowing difficulty has been identified.

- Provide assistance:

  - Check that chunks of food eaten are not too large. Pre-cut the food before serving if needed.

  - If providing feeding assistance check the food is swallowed and the mouth is empty before offering more food.

- Enhance familiarity:

    - Present favourite foods to prevent the spitting out of food and, once eating, offer the original meal or further foods.

    - Consider using culturally familiar foods to help its recognition.

- Socialisation:

    - Try eating your meal with the person. Eating with company can enhance mealtime abilities owing to social interaction and taking cues to eat from others.

- Adjust environment:

    - Introduce relaxing music to suit the person's preferences. Negative environmental influences at mealtimes include visual overstimulation in a crowded room and auditory confusion secondary to background noise. Adjusting one or more of these negative environmental influences may improve behaviour.

- REFERRAL: If the spitting out of food persists, liaise with an SLP/SLT for further advice.

5. Reduced ability chewing

- IMPORTANT NOTICE: If the reduced ability to chew is thought to compromise someone's safety (i.e. you witness signs of aspiration) when eating or drinking, liaise with a speech and language pathologist/therapist (SLP/SLT) immediately.

- IMPORTANT NOTICE: If the reduced ability for chewing is secondary to fatigue, refer to an SLP/SLT and offer smaller, more frequent meals throughout the day to reduce fatigue at mealtimes.

- Check oral health:

    - Check for inadequate or missing dentition, loose dentures or sores, ulcers and broken teeth.

- Provide cueing:
  - Use verbal prompting to remind the person when to chew.
  - Use manual prompting and visual 'modelling' by demonstrating chewing so the person can imitate.
  - Try manual prompting by applying light pressure on the lips or under the chin to stimulate chewing.
  - Manually prompt the person by presenting an empty spoon or fork back up towards the mouth, as if you are offering the next mouthful, as this may remind the person to chew.

- Adapt food:
  - Offer smaller bites of foods moistened by gravies or sauces if no swallowing difficulty has been identified.

- Texture modification:
  - Trial a different food texture by providing softer foods that are easier to chew and swallow. Use the Dysphagia Diet Food Texture Descriptors or IDDSI Framework and Descriptors to define the correct soft consistency if a swallowing difficulty has been identified.
  - Transitioning to a soft or purée diet may be indicated and should be advised by an SLP/SLT. Use the Dysphagia Diet Food Texture Descriptors or IDDSI Framework and Descriptors to define the correct soft or thickened purée consistency if a swallowing difficulty has been identified.

- Provide assistance:
  - Try offering small bites of food one at a time if providing assistance with eating.

- REFERRAL: If the reduced ability to chew persists, liaise with an SLP/SLT for further advice.

6. Prolonged chewing without swallowing

- IMPORTANT NOTICE: If the prolonged chewing without swallowing is thought to compromise someone's safety (i.e.

you witness signs of aspiration) when eating or drinking, liaise with a speech and language pathologist/therapist (SLP/SLT) immediately.

- Check oral health:
  - Check for inadequate or missing dentition, loose dentures or sores, ulcers and broken teeth.

- Provide cueing:
  - Use verbal prompting to remind the person when to swallow.
  - Once you have noticed that the person has chewed the food adequately, use verbal prompting to remind them to swallow.
  - Use manual prompting and 'modelling' to demonstrate swallowing so the person can imitate.
  - Manually prompt the person by presenting an empty spoon or fork back up towards the mouth, as if you are offering the next mouthful, as this may remind them to swallow.
  - Manually prompting the person by stroking their throat gently can encourage swallowing.

- Adapt food:
  - Offer smaller bites of foods moistened by gravies or sauces if no swallowing difficulty has been identified.

- Sensory adaptation:
  - Try alternating temperature and taste within meals, for example warm stewed apple with ice-cream, or curry with yoghurt, if no swallowing difficulty has been identified.
  - Trial food appetisers with heightened sensory input, for example salty, cold, sweet, sharp, carbonated, spicy or crunchy. Alternate between different foods to encourage the person to start eating. Use the Dysphagia Diet Food Texture Descriptors or IDDSI Framework and Descriptors to

define the correct food consistency if a swallowing difficulty has been identified.

- Offering teaspoons or sips of ice-cold drinks before and during a meal will stimulate stronger swallows and help to clear remaining oral residue. Thickened fluids may be required if a swallowing difficulty has been identified; use the Dysphagia Diet Food Texture Descriptors or IDDSI Framework and Descriptors to define the correct consistency.

• Texture modification:

- Trial a different food texture by providing softer foods that are easier to chew and swallow. Use the Dysphagia Diet Food Texture Descriptors or IDDSI Framework and Descriptors to define the correct soft consistency if a swallowing difficulty has been identified.

- Transitioning to a soft or purée diet may be indicated and should be advised on by an SLP/SLT. Use the Dysphagia Diet Food Texture Descriptors or IDDSI Framework and Descriptors to define the correct soft or thickened purée consistency if a swallowing difficulty has been identified.

• REFERRAL: If the prolonged chewing without swallowing persists, liaise with an SLP/SLT for further advice.

7. Does not chew food before swallowing

• IMPORTANT NOTICE: If choking is a hazard or not chewing food before swallowing is thought to compromise someone's safety (i.e. you witness signs of aspiration) when eating or drinking, liaise with a speech and language pathologist/therapist (SLP/SLT) immediately.

• Check oral health:

- Check for inadequate or missing dentition, loose dentures or sores, ulcers and broken teeth.

- Provide cueing:

  - Use verbal prompting to remind the person to chew before swallowing.

  - Use manual prompting and visual 'modelling' by demonstrating chewing so the person can imitate.

- Socialisation:

  - Try eating your meal with the person. Eating with company can enhance mealtime abilities owing to social interaction and taking cues to eat from others.

- Texture modification:

  - Trial a different food texture by providing softer foods that are easier to chew and swallow. Use the Dysphagia Diet Food Texture Descriptors or IDDSI Framework and Descriptors to define the correct soft consistency if a swallowing difficulty has been identified.

  - Transitioning to a soft or purée diet may be indicated and should be advised on by an SLP/SLT. Use the Dysphagia Diet Food Texture Descriptors or IDDSI Framework and Descriptors to define the correct soft or thickened purée consistency if a swallowing difficulty has been identified.

- REFERRAL: If the abscence of chewing food before swallowing persists, liaise with an SLP/SLT for further advice.

8. Reduced ability swallowing or refusing to swallow

- IMPORTANT NOTICE: If you suspect the person has a swallowing difficulty (i.e. you witness signs of aspiration) or is consistently refusing to swallow please liaise with a speech and language pathologist/therapist (SLP/SLT) immediately.

- Check oral health:

  - Check for inadequate or missing dentition, loose dentures or sores, ulcers and broken teeth.

- Provide cueing:
  - Use verbal prompting to remind the person to swallow with each bite.
  - Manually prompting the person by stroking their throat gently can encourage swallowing.
  - Manually prompt the person by presenting an empty spoon or fork back up towards the mouth, as if you are offering the next mouthful, as this may remind them to swallow.
  - Softly stroking the person's arm or using calming rhythmic patting and talking to them about the food can help swallowing if refusal is seen.
- Adapt food:
  - Offer smaller bites of foods moistened by gravies or sauces if no swallowing difficulty has been identified.
- Sensory adaptation:
  - Trial food appetisers with heightened sensory input, for example salty, cold, sweet, sharp, carbonated, spicy or crunchy. Alternate between different foods to encourage the person to start eating. Use the Dysphagia Diet Food Texture Descriptors or IDDSI Framework and Descriptors to define the correct food consistency if a swallowing difficulty has been identified.
- Enhance familiarity:
  - The person may benefit from receiving assistance, recognising the voice from one specific carer or have consistency in caring (and feeding) practices. With advancing dementia people need to recognise their carers or somehow realise they are there to assist with eating.
  - Ask if a family member can help to encourage the person to eat.

- Socialisation:

    - Try eating your meal with the person. Eating with company can enhance mealtime abilities owing to social interaction and taking cues to eat from others.

- Provide assistance:

    - Try offering small bites of food one at a time if providing assistance with eating.

- Adjust environment:

    - Negative environmental influences at mealtimes include visual overstimulation in a crowded room and auditory confusion secondary to background noise. Adjusting one or more of these negative environmental influences may improve behaviour.

- REFERRAL: If the reduced ability to swallow or refusing to swallow persists, liaise with an SLP/SLT for further advice.

10

Meal Behaviours

EFFECT OF THE MEALTIME ENVIRONMENT

Introduction: the mealtime environment

The physical environment at a mealtime environment can make eating one of the most challenging activities of daily living for older people living with dementia. It is impossible to say what the most significant feature of mealtime care should be to improve nutrition and hydration but the environment interacts with everything that takes place at a mealtime and is perhaps one of the most important aspects. Throughout the preceding chapters, interventions that have involved changes to aspects of the mealtime environment have been related to specific reduced mealtime abilities. For example in Chapter 4 if someone has 'Reduced ability in identifying food from plate' then interventions improving the colour contrast of the tableware and table setting as well as providing optimum lighting are suggested. Many of the interventions previously discussed are also required to help provide a more supportive mealtime environment and reduce meal behaviours that affect food intake. Therefore although this chapter will introduce new concepts to improve the mealtime environment, it will also refer to what has been discussed in previous chapters.

It is worth noting that there are interventions based slightly outside of the mealtime environment that may also impact on improved nutrition and hydration and/or meal behaviours. These include interventions that increase social interactions through food-based activities such as breakfast clubs or using improved wayfinding techniques to help orientate the person with dementia in the right direction (Whear *et al.*, 2014), but these are not fully discussed in this book as the focus is on the mealtime environment.

There are many aspects of the mealtime environment that can inhibit the abilities of a person with dementia to eat and drink. Providing an unsupportive mealtime setting where it is difficult to see, pick up and eat the food will make the tasks necessary for eating and drinking very difficult. Research indicates that those with middle-stage dementia exposed to a supportive mealtime environment do not experience the same level of reduced eating abilities as those in an unsupportive one (Slaughter *et al.*, 2011).

It is therefore necessary to enhance the abilities of someone living with dementia by providing a supportive mealtime setting. Simple environmental interventions can improve nutritional intake and preserve or enhance mealtime eating abilities (Chaudhury *et al.*, 2013). By modifying the mealtime environment and making it more 'dementia friendly' it is arguable that you will also improve the meal experience and enhance quality of life.

Why the environment affects eating abilities and behaviours in people living with dementia

The full range of senses needs to be considered when creating a supportive mealtime setting. People living with dementia have increased dependence on their senses and two senses are highly impacted by the mealtime environment: sight (vision) which is stimulated by light, and hearing which is stimulated by sound/noise.

Loss of hearing can affect 40 per cent of people over 65 years of age. Hearing loss is related to a decline in cognition and impacts behavioural symptoms of dementia although the exact reasons for this are not clear and will involve numerous factors (Hardy *et al.*, 2016). Noise is a major source of sensory stimulation and for people living with dementia overstimulation by noise can have negative effects causing auditory confusion, disorientation, agitation, loss of balance and decreased quality of life (SCIE, 2015b).

Aside from overstimulation a reduced perception of sound can cause cortical deafness, 'word deafness', auditory agnosia and auditory hallucinations. This means the person experiences increased difficulty identifying or understanding sounds, for example not recognising a familiar voice when background noise is loud, or not understanding a request from someone with an unfamiliar accent (Hardy *et al.*, 2016).

Hearing loss or not wearing a hearing aid can compound these problems (Brush and Calkins, 2008).

Loss of sight affects 123,000 people with dementia according to the RNIB Scotland. Causes of sight loss include cataracts and other eye conditions, various health problems and normal ageing of the eye. People with dementia can also experience difficulties perceiving what they see rather than how sharply they see, despite having healthy eyes. This may be a reason for a change in behaviour seen at mealtimes, for example seeming confused and disoriented, becoming withdrawn or uncommunicative or finding it hard to locate food on the plate (RNIB Scotland, 2012). The RNIB Scotland have a useful 'Identifying sight loss' checklist which includes symptoms to look out for at mealtimes including observing if the person knocks over items, leaves food on the plate or searches for objects with their hands (RNIB Scotland, 2012). The difficulty in getting a diagnosis related to visual problems affected by dementia and how this shapes your sensory environment has been highlighted by Agnes Houston MBE. Agnes lives well with dementia and from interviewing other people living with dementia has produced a useful booklet on dementia and sensory challenges which is freely available (Life Changes Trust, 2015).

The other sense that is impacted at mealtimes is the sense of smell; ways to improve or adapt a declining smell and taste have been discussed in Chapter 6 and will not be repeated here.

It is usually not possible to significantly medically improve conditions related to vision and hearing, therefore practical interventions are required but are often overlooked. It is important that these senses are stimulated and supported in the right way to provide additional cues to help someone understand they are in a mealtime environment and that it is time to eat (Timlin and Rysenbry, 2010). Hearing loss and visual impairment associated with dementia and ageing, in combination with increased agitation and confusion, can mean a mealtime environment will provide high levels of stimulation which someone living with dementia may find difficult to filter and make sense of. Similarly if the environment before or during the mealtime is devoid of any sensory stimulation the person with dementia may exhibit signs of apathy or decreased alertness, or it may cause someone to be more impatient (Department of Health, 2015). Indeed restlessness and agitation have been observed affecting up to 93 per cent of people living with dementia in care home settings (Chaudhury et al., 2013).

If the environment is not supportive then the person with dementia may display these and other behaviours at mealtimes. A list of the most common observed meal behaviours is provided below and interventions to support these behaviours are detailed in the following practical interventions chapter. These behaviours impact the ability of someone living with dementia to eat and maintain adequate nutritional intake. Since carers may observe any number of multiple meal behaviours they need to have interventions readily at hand to provide support to each individual's behaviours.

Common meal behaviours that can impact on nutritional intake and affect quality of life

- Hoards, hides, throws or plays with food

- Eats other people's food (or drink)

- Refuses to eat (verbally or physically)

- Bats away or pushes away spoon presented by carer

- Turns head away when being fed

- Distracted from eating

- Demonstrates impatient behaviour around mealtimes

- Eats small amounts and leaves table

- Walks during mealtime or unable to sit still for meals

- Shows agitated behaviour or irritability

Adapted from Durnbaugh et al. (1996); Crawley and Hocking (2011)

The definition and term 'meal behaviours' was discussed in Chapter 2 as part of the range of mealtime abilities often observed in people with dementia. Meal behaviours are distressing and often interrupt or prevent eating for not only the person experiencing them but also other people with dementia in the same mealtime environment (Gilmore-Bykovskyi, 2015). The acceptance in dementia care is that behaviours are the person's way of responding to an environment or situation that is not supporting their current level of cognition (Chaudhury et al., 2013). A change in their behaviour is a symptom of this but may also be seen as a form of communication. One author famously described these behaviours as 'unmet needs', which is a term that has stuck and was discussed previously in Chapter 2.

By manipulating the environment using relatively simple modifications you can reduce the cognitive demands placed on a person, helping to reduce meal behaviours and allow eating abilities to be preserved or enhanced. An unsupportive environment is one of the most common concerns mentioned by carers in nursing homes (Chaudhury *et al.*, 2013), while the environment in acute settings has also been identified by nurses as a major factor affecting nutritional intake (Walton *et al.*, 2013).

This chapter will therefore focus on evidence-based interventions to create a supportive mealtime environment and relate these interventions to enhancing the observed common meal behaviours listed previously.

The evidence for adjusting the mealtime environment

The evidence section in this chapter will be split to discuss unsupportive and supportive environmental influences at mealtimes. The majority of research looking at environmental modifications to the mealtime is based in residential care; however, many of the interventions or principles of the interventions can be applied to a home care or acute care setting.

Assessing the mealtime environment

Many things need to be considered when providing a supportive environment for people with dementia, and to help with this a short summary of practical tools used in the assessment of the mealtime environment follows.

There are many assessment tools freely available to help both home care and care homes create a more supportive mealtime environment. These tools are not solely confined to the mealtime but encompass the whole of the living environment and provide general recommendations. If you wish to audit the mealtime or living environment of the persons with dementia you care for, then the two internet-based resources below will provide both simple and very detailed starting points.

1. **EHE Environmental Assessment Tool** (The King's Fund, 2014) This assessment tool has seven sections with section 3 focused on the mealtime environment. It is a simple and basic tool that covers the main 'dementia-friendly' environmental themes.

2. **Dementia Care Environment Audit Tools and Services** (DEEP, 2015a) The Australian-based Dementia Enabling Environments Project (DEEP) provides access to several very detailed audit tools that cover care homes, gardens and communities as well as additional information on specific aspects of the environment such as lighting.

Apart from simple or detailed audit tools there are also two excellent resources that include an interactive picture diagram of a dining environment, and other living environments, which can be found on the websites below. As you click on the objects in the dining room an explanation of how to modify that aspect is presented.

- Produced in association with Alzheimer's Australia the 'Dementia Enabling Environments' website is available online (DEEP, 2015b).[1]

- Based in the UK at the University of Sterling the Dementia Services Development Centre (DSDC) has produced a 'Virtual Environments' section on their website (DSDC, 2012b).[2]

Unsupportive environment

An unsupportive environment can trigger the symptoms of dementia, increasing agitation, irritability, apathy and confusion (Dewing, 2009). Unsupportive environments can also contribute to malnutrition and associated ill health and make any caring duties at mealtimes more complex (Chaudhury *et al.*, 2013). This final point could lead to carers feeling the person with dementia is resisting or refusing care and/ or food. It is worth being aware of common mealtime environmental aspects that could be considered unsupportive to the person with dementia as displayed in Table 10.1. Interestingly unsupportive dining environments are one of the most voiced concerns of carers in nursing homes (Chaudhury *et al.*, 2013).

---

1   www.enablingenvironments.com.au
2   http://dementia.stir.ac.uk/design/virtual-environments/virtual-care-home

Table 10.1: Summary of unsupportive environmental influences at mealtimes

Environmental influences	Unsupportive environmental aspects that can inhibit mealtime abilities
Noise levels (Auditory distractions can provide unwanted stimulation)	Sitting near a corridor or serving path, a window with noise outside, having loud dining companions, background noises (telephones ringing, machines beeping, staff activity, kitchen noise, trolleys, people coming and going, etc.) and inappropriate radio or TV stations during the mealtime can all contribute to unsupportive auditory stimulation and can become overwhelming
Lighting levels (Insufficient lighting can affect the ability to visually clarify items on the table and/or the food)	*Natural light*: Although windows can let in additional light especially at midday (lunch tends to be the main meal of the day) this can cause unwanted glare as light is reflected from shiny or polished fixtures (tables), fittings (floors, glossy walls, doors) and tableware (plastic tablecloths). Additionally some people may not want to sit by a window, while others may enjoy this *Artificial light*: Where light fixtures are positioned affects visual clarity. For example if the dining room only has one central light it will cause the perimeters to be dimmer, meaning those eating in the corners of the room will have lower levels of light
Tableware (A lack of visual colour contrast makes it harder to clarify items)	Finding it hard to see the plates, cutlery, fluid in cups or food on the plate can all be affected by a lack of visual contrast. For example white plates and white tablecloth with silver cutlery provide very low contrast (making it difficult to identify the plate from the table), while the cutlery blends into the tablecloth (making it harder to spot). Similarly a highly patterned tablecloth or plate can cause the same effect, making food hard to recognise
Socialisation and stimulation (With whom and where someone is positioned at mealtimes can have a negative influence on behaviour)	*Overstimulation*: Sitting in a busy or crowded area of the dining room (e.g. the centre), with staff milling around serving others, can feel crowded and noisy; being positioned next to the corridor or entrance to the dining room can be especially noisy and busy – causing excess stimulation. Being seated next to someone who is displaying meal behaviours may also be overstimulating. Regarding personal preferences it is worth remembering that the person may be used to eating alone or with only one other person and may feel overstimulated in a group dining environment. Avoid an institutional appearance and patterned walls and carpets *Understimulation*: Sitting for a long time with nothing to do before food is served can be understimulating and may cause a loss of interest in eating. This may become more apparent in people who are not seated with friends or those they have an affinity with

Carer interaction (This occurs at the mealtime and including when providing feeding assistance)	A rigid and task-orientated mealtime does not seem to benefit those living with dementia. The carer's beliefs and knowledge on how dementia affects mealtime abilities can also influence food consumption. Organisational rules and culture can impact negatively on carers. Finally if the carer is experiencing stress when providing feeding assistance this may negatively affect the food intake of the person with dementia. See text for more detail

Adapted from Brush (2001); Brush et al. (2002); Brush and Calkins (2008); Dewing (2009); Chaudhury et al. (2013); Whear et al. (2014); SCIE (2015b); Woodbridge et al. (2018)

Carer interaction

Previous research has shown that carer interaction can influence the amount of food consumed, with a better quality of interaction increasing the food intake (Amella, 1999). Researchers looking at the interaction between care staff and those with 'aversive feeding behaviours' – or meal behaviours as this book prefers – have identified some interesting themes. One revolves around the common meal behaviour in people with severe dementia of refusing food, in whom this behaviour is seen more often (Pasman et al., 2003). It seems some carers interpreted an increase in food refusal meal behaviours as a loss of interest in food and after a couple of times stopped any further attempts to support the person to eat and drink; whereas other carers saw the food refusal as part of a range of reduced mealtime abilities that required further support, and they continued to help but with different interventions (Pasman et al., 2003). The most interesting discovery in this research was that both of these carers' interactions were observed on the same person with dementia. This meant that when one type of carer would stop providing assistance, the other would continue to try different supportive interventions, leading to the same person having better or worse food intake depending on how the carer interpreted the food refusal meal behaviour. Worryingly the carers never communicated with each other or detailed in any care plans what interventions may have been successful in the people they were caring for. For example one of the common meal behaviours listed at the start of this chapter is 'Bats away or pushes away spoon presented by carer'. In this study when this meal behaviour was observed some of the carers stopped providing feeding assistance because they interpreted this rejection as the person not wanting to live any more. Other carers thought that it was because of a fear of choking, as the person had a swallowing difficulty, while still other carers thought the person did not recognise the food.

This type of situation can occur every day in care for people with later-stage dementia. What the true reason is for food refusal often can never be known, as unfortunately it can be impossible to communicate this. Therefore the carer's perception of the food refusal dictates whether further support is provided (Watson, 2003). Carers are facing an ethical decision each time they witness meal behaviours such as this; should they continue to feed or stop feeding (Watson, 2003)? Refusal to eat is often observed in those with later-stage dementia and can cause a range of ethical considerations (unfortunately outside the remit of this book). Carers are often unable to distinguish between a lack of mealtime abilities or desire to eat, or a plain refusal to eat, making it impossible to know if the reason for 'refusal' is an unwillingness to eat, a lack of understanding regarding the cues related to eating, or a severe reduction in the abilities required to eat and drink (Watson, 1996).

Perhaps for some people with dementia they no longer wish to eat and they independently choose not to eat as they find it too complex. As a carer you assume they do want to eat and a combination of cognitive decline, the mealtime environment and preserved eating abilities all affect sufficient food intake. It is important that when a person is refusing to eat, all possible interventions to provide better support for reduced mealtime abilities are first implemented and assessed for effectiveness.

Additionally carers can encourage meal behaviours unknowingly via their caring interactions. For example agitation can be increased when offering food to eat too quickly; or if the person with dementia is ignored then agitation can increase along with attention at mealtimes. Resistance to care can also be seen when physical or verbal controlling techniques are used by carers at mealtimes. This can happen when the carer is struggling to provide effective feeding assistance and the meal is dominated by task-focused instructions rather than including person-centred interactions (Gilmore-Bykovskyi, 2015).

A rigid and task-orientated mealtime does not seem to benefit those living with dementia, as individual preferences and needs are not adapted to (Mamhidir et al., 2007). Carers who are observed to seem 'bothered' or 'inflexible' lead to an increase in meal behaviours (Aselage et al., 2011). On the plus side when training is provided and carers understand the mealtime abilities and behaviours associated with dementia they themselves are more supportive and eating has been shown to improve (Mamhidir *et al.*, 2007)

Carer stress

This loss of being able to feed oneself and reliance on assistance can increase the burden placed on carers (Chang and Roberts, 2008). The deterioration seen in the person living with dementia at a mealtime who is experiencing a range of reduced mealtime abilities has been shown to be a source of stress and burden for the carer whether they are paid or unpaid (Rivière *et al.*, 2002). The task of managing mealtime abilities can be daunting to both family carer and professionals (Aselage *et al.*, 2011). Nurses caring for these individuals have reported feeding residents as one of the most difficult daily management problems (Watson, 1996). Nursing staff have also expressed feelings of 'helplessness' when trying to provide mealtime assistance to those with reduced mealtime abilities and increased meal behaviours (Mamhidir *et al.*, 2007).

Some carers have felt that to care for people with dementia at mealtimes is to do the 'undoable' (Hammar, Swall and Meranius, 2016). They have struggled between doing what they think is best for the person within the confines of the organisational structure they have to work in. Carers have also felt stress over making decisions regarding whether the person wishes to eat, after they observe food refusal. As discussed above this ethical dilemma led them to feelings of guilt over whether they had made the right decision: to stop feeding assistance or to continue? Furthermore providing less assistance to those who were a bit more independent, as more support was provided to others with less independence, led carers to worry if these people had eaten enough (Hammar *et al.*, 2016). Many of the issues raised by Hammar and colleagues could be directly related to organisational issues such as lack of staff or lack of support for staff, with carers feeling abandoned by seniors. Lack of knowledge by carers on how to support people with dementia at mealtimes who display reduced mealtime abilities was also a factor. But not being able to implement interventions owing to organisational constraints was an additional negative factor regardless of the carer's level of knowledge. It is clearly impossible for carers to provide person-centred care in this type of work environment and yet it is a common occurrence. If an organisation sees mealtime care for people with dementia as 'basic care' rather than one of the most complex caring duties then nutrition and hydration will never be a priority. Indeed as Hammar and colleagues (2016) rightly say, a lack of organisational support at mealtimes may violate the dignity of the person with dementia and may be observed as a betrayal of their care needs.

Overwhelming noise levels attributed to staff activities

The quality of carer interactions with the people they care for can also be impacted by their job responsibilities. One major source of noise is the activities of staff (talking, telephone ringing, doors slamming, alarm sounding, noisy movement, etc.) (Dewing, 2009) with even low-level background noise (that carers hardly notice) causing distress in some individuals with dementia (SCIE, 2015b). It can be difficult for carers to identify their normal activity as noise; however, if someone is displaying an increase in meal behaviours at mealtimes then noise from caring activities and staff should be considered as a potential factor. An assessment or audit of background noises that occur at a mealtime and how this affects those with dementia may be indicated to help identify improvements (SCIE, 2015b).

Supportive environment

A supportive environment can compensate for the reduction or loss of sight and/or hearing and also augment the effects of interventions implemented to support other reduced mealtime abilities. Importantly a supportive mealtime environment can provide additional cues to eat and also enhance the ability of the carer to provide assistance if needed and at the appropriate levels. Mealtime environmental aspects that could be considered supportive to the person with dementia are shown in Table 10.2 and described in this section.

Table 10.2: Summary of practical interventions to
provide a supportive mealtime environment

Environmental interventions	Environmental aspects that can support behaviours at mealtimes
Noise reduction and enhancement plus use of music (Too much noise is overstimulating but appropriate noise can be calming)	To reduce the general noise in a dining room the sound needs to be absorbed rather than bounced around the room. Include sound-absorbent materials such as plain coloured carpets, cork floors or rugs; curtains or drapes for windows are simple modifications. Acoustic panels can be added to walls and can provide an old-fashioned panel effect

To reduce noise from carers, first the carers need to recognise they make noise (see the text for carer interactions). Stop any non-mealtime activities such as cleaning or vacuuming

Music can decrease aggression or anxiety. Suitable music choices could include classical, jazz/big band, easy listening, popular music from the 1950–1970s or any ambient music from a suitable era. More popular recent music genres are generally not familiar and may be distracting (or indeed annoying) |
| **Optimum lighting** (It is important to achieve a balance between artificial light and natural light if possible, while avoiding glare) | *Natural light*: Make the most of and enhance natural light but avoid glare. Natural light needs to be softened and filtered through blinds or textiles. Install sheer curtains or paper shades to deflect glare while letting light in. Avoid blinds which do block glare but also block desirable natural light. Prevent glare off table surfaces by using tablecloths or coverings on reflective floors

Artificial light: Dining room light should be evenly distributed but still reduce glare. Conceal artificial light sources (bulbs) with light fittings to reduce glare or use cove lights and other indirect lighting such as 'uplights' rather than lights directing down. Add wall lighting in less-well-lit areas like in corners of rooms to illuminate the meal setting and prevent glare. Additional indirect overhead lighting may be required in other less-well-lit areas like the middle of a larger dining room |
| **Tableware and colour contrast** (ensure a high visual colour contrast) | Attention to food can increase through visual cues, such as ensuring visual contrast between plate, food and place setting. For example a dark blue tablecloth and white plate with silver cutlery provide high contrast, making identifying/seeing the plate and cutlery much easier. The colour of the plate does not always have to change. Presenting a variety of coloured foods in attractive ways helps identify the food from the white plate. Ensuring optimum lighting at the mealtime can also enhance the colour contrast of tableware used. Tableware, contrast and lighting are discussed in detail in Chapter 4 along with a summary table of different tableware contrast designs |

cont.

Environmental interventions	Environmental aspects that can support behaviours at mealtimes
Socialisation and stimulation during mealtime (A positive social environment can promote the mealtime abilities and behaviours of people with dementia)	Supporting an individual's preferred level of social interaction with others can help reduce meal behaviours caused by under- or overstimulation of the senses Consider appropriate seating arrangements based on relative need, social compatibility and personalities of individuals rather than comparable levels of independence/dependence. Provide small tables that encourage conversation among tablemates. Round tables encourage interaction and may be suitable for some, whereas square tables help define boundaries which will be more appropriate for others Avoid seating people long before the meal is ready Stimulation in a busy dining room can be reduced by creating space and privacy using moveable dividers. Serving people with dementia in smaller dining rooms if available can minimise distractions
Carer interaction (This can directly affect food intake)	The carer's interactions include touch and voice and can be very important as people with dementia may need additional cues to recognise their carers. If someone prefers receiving assistance from a particular carer observe how they interact and care for the person to help identify supportive mealtime strategies and record this in a care plan
Homelike settings (These provide a sense of familiarity)	A more homelike mealtime environment can help provide cues to eating and drinking and reduce meal behaviours. Minimise the institutional or non-dining-room appearance of a mealtime environment by removing equipment, garbage, laundry and so on when not in use Use fixtures to create a homelike environment such as chandeliers, plants, formal window treatments, hanging artwork or a low-profile table centrepiece, for example flowers in a vase Try using an eclectic mix of furniture (avoid patterned styles) that does not have to match, as coordinated furniture can look more institutionalised. Ensure plain or unpatterned or low-contrast pattern flooring/carpet is used and avoid flooring that is highly reflective The style of service can also provide more familiarity and increase social interaction, for example self-service at the table like a traditional family dinner meal rather than pre-plated food served by the carer, or consuming your meal with the person

Adapted from Brush (2001); Brush *et al.* (2002); Brush and Calkins (2008); Dewing (2009); Chaudhury *et al.* (2013); Whear *et al.* (2014); SCIE (2015b); Woodbridge *et al.* (2018)

Auditory interventions

NOISE REDUCTION AND ENHANCEMENT

For those with increased sensitivity to sound and/or hearing loss practical modifications to reduce the noise in the environment along with employing clever strategies for communication can be effective interventions. Examples of communication interventions include using written communication aids and pictorial or electronic devices, ensuring face-to-face communication is free of overwhelming background noise and avoiding sounds that cause distress. To enhance hearing then, hearing aids or other hearing assistive devices and also earwax removal can help improve hearing deficits and activities of daily living too (Hardy *et al.*, 2016).

Table 10.2 provides suggestions for ways to reduce noise in the mealtime environment by modifying furniture and fittings in the room while also being aware of unwanted noise caused by staff or non-mealtime activities. Media sounds (television, radio, music) can all provide meaningful stimulation at mealtimes (see music in the supportive influences section); however, there will be those who are not interested in the media and others it affects negatively. All these types of media can create excess background noise, making it more difficult for someone with dementia and those with hearing impairments to focus on the mealtime. As a general rule television is usually best turned off for mealtimes; the preferred types of music are discussed in the supportive section below. Remember that although a TV or radio can provide welcome stimulation to one person it can be a source of unwanted noise to another.

MUSIC AT MEALTIMES

The therapeutic use of music (music therapy) both can reduce agitation (Sung and Chang, 2005) and has the potential to increase social interaction and improve physical functioning of people with dementia (O'Neil *et al.*, 2011). Music played in the background during activities can improve mood, and even memory, and helps the person to engage (Jakob and Collier, 2013).

If music can therefore be applied to a mealtime setting and enhance mealtime abilities then the benefits should be noticeable. Also, listening to music during mealtimes is a simple, low-cost and feasible intervention option. Unfortunately despite some positive research, in general the true effect of recorded music at mealtimes is still debatable. A Cochrane systematic review indicated a lack of evidence to prove using music is any more effective than not using music (Vink *et al.*, 2004), while a more recent review also highlights many methodological issues with the current research (O'Neil *et al.*, 2011) making it hard to draw firm conclusions.

A limited amount of research however has shown some positive benefit of playing certain types of music at mealtimes, in the short term at least. For example more food may be consumed and agitation may reduce when classical and/or soothing music is played while eating (Engstrom and Marmstal Hammar, 2012). Soft jazz, romantic or 'elevator music' (without words) without sudden changes in tempo or volume may also be a suitable option (Ragneskog *et al.*, 1996). Several studies have shown a beneficial effect of music at mealtimes on aggressive behaviour and agitation, and to a lesser extent on hiding/hoarding items (Whear *et al.*, 2014). If music is to be used to improve mealtime behaviour or food intake then it is worth considering that if the person is not exhibiting any signs of agitation/aggressive behaviour then perhaps the addition of music will not have a significant impact.

Other benefits of music may include spending more time at the mealtime. If an individual seems restless, demonstrates impatience and often leaves the table then this may be an approach to adopt to help alleviate the behaviour (Ragneskog *et al.*, 1996).

One of the main limitations with the research looking at music interventions is the unknown effect this has had on the staff, with several studies (Ragneskog *et al.*, 1996; O'Neil *et al.*, 2011; Chaudhury *et al.*, 2013) being unsure whether the changes in eating abilities and meal behaviour were seen because of the effects of music or the staff being more attentive. For example in one study where the amount of food eaten was found to increase in the group receiving music as an intervention, the care staff actually served more food (Ragneskog *et al.*, 1996). Therefore the increased food intake could not be clearly separated from the fact that the people with dementia had received more food on their plates (O'Neil *et al.*, 2011).

Factors like this may be unwanted variables in research but not in the real world of dementia care. If music improves staff mood, or helps them concentrate, or whatever it does in making them provide more supportive care then this is a positive outcome for both the person with dementia and carer. There are some practical points that need to be considered before trialling or adopting music as an intervention at mealtimes:

- When choosing a type of music it is best to ask the person their preferences and create a list of liked or appropriate listening choices. There are now many reminiscence software applications or life story works that could help with this. In a group-living setting it would be best if everyone could come to an agreement although this may be impossible.

- If the person with dementia cannot indicate their musical preferences then carers should consider their age, interest and other media-viewing habits to help determine the most appropriate music. Clearly family members can also provide insight.

- Whatever music is chosen it will need to be monitored regularly and this is especially important in group living where other people are affected. What one person finds relaxing the other may find unbearably annoying. For example music that increases meal behaviours such as agitation or distractions in others should be avoided. Or if a negative change or a decrease in eating abilities is observed then music as an intervention will need to be reassessed for that person. 'Soft' background music may sound pleasant to some, especially if they have good hearing, but it may sound like noise or static to someone with a hearing impairment.

- The main reason for introducing music should be to produce a relaxing atmosphere and reduce signs of agitation, aggression or distraction in an individual. It can also add to creating a pleasant environment for both carer and the person with dementia.

- Ensure the sound level is audible and pleasant for both the person with dementia and the carer; it may need to be adjusted throughout the mealtime depending on the type and quality of media used.

- Finally use music at mealtimes for a set period of time; for example start half an hour before, and continue during and for half an hour after the mealtime, thus giving a purpose to using music. Research has looked at different lengths of time but what seems best is to start just before the mealtime and continue until the last person has finished eating (Ragneskog *et al.*, 1996).

The evidence around therapeutic use of music also includes singing; however, clearly the use of singing at mealtimes may cause problems, for example singing rather than eating or the potential risk of choking in those with swallowing difficulties. This is not to say that singing as part of other activities will not contribute to improved eating abilities at mealtimes. Observations from charities (Sing For Your Life, 2014) using this approach claim some success with improved appetite but there is no research from which to make recommendations.

A HUMMING CASE STUDY

Interestingly another intervention option for carers is humming songs while providing full feeding assistance at mealtimes. In a case study of only two people with severe dementia the carers hummed while feeding over two weeks with positive effects of improving mealtime eating abilities in one woman but no difference in eating abilities in the other (Engstrom and Marmstal Hammar, 2012). A study on two people where the intervention did not work on one of them is hardly conclusive. As the authors mention, the woman who reacted positively may have simply preferred or enjoyed the songs being hummed while the other did not, or may have had worsening symptoms on the days she was observed. Nevertheless there is very limited evidence on successful interventions for feeding people with severe dementia who are refusing to eat or experiencing other meal behaviours. A cost-free intervention of humming may be a useful caring technique to support some individuals requiring full feeding assistance.

Optimum lighting

Older adults require more light for clarity of vision with a thickening and yellowing of the lens of the eye and decreased pupil size reducing the amount of light received (Brush, 2001). As an older retina takes in less light older people can require two to four times the amount of light to see satisfactorily compared to younger people (Brush and Calkins, 2008; DSDC, 2012a). Decreased pupil reaction time and less elasticity of the lens can also cause increased sensitivity to glare from light sources and decrease the ability to adapt quickly to changing light levels (Timlin and Rysenbry, 2010). Appropriate lighting should therefore prevent glare, avoid shadows and balance ambient light to help compensate for poor eyesight and enhance the ability to see and eat food.

The light in dining rooms is recommended to be at a level of 300 lux (a unit of illumination) from artificial lighting or daylight (DEEP, 2015c). This can be measured with a light meter but obtaining accurate results may be difficult and a professional may be required to assess this. Changing the light in a dining room to make it more suitable for people with dementia is relatively easy and cheap to accomplish.

Dim lighting may exaggerate visual problems and the person may observe the food, plate, table items and utensils as appearing to blend together. It is important to maximise the use of natural light (sunlight) as it is more dispersed and lights a larger area — therefore providing higher levels of light than electric lightbulbs. Older people however are also more sensitive to glare, meaning any increase in lighting must be considered appropriately. Glare can be distracting to a person with dementia and often presents in a dining room in two forms:

1. direct glare, which comes from inadequately shielded light sources and must be avoided, for example sunlight through a large window

2. reflected glare, which is created by strong light bouncing off smooth, reflective surfaces like shiny tables.

Both types and large amounts of glare can make seeing the plate and food on the table a lot more challenging. Therefore although more light may be needed, too much light can still cause vision problems if it causes glare. Table 10.2 provides some practical ideas on how to prevent glare at mealtimes from both natural and artificial light. Typically there are issues with sub-optimum lighting in a home or care home: uneven light levels, the person with dementia has difficulty reading the menu, very little natural light is available, glare is coming from the windows, light bulbs have varying colour renditions and ceiling lights cause glare on the tables and/or pictures on the walls.

Tableware and contrast

For the practical purpose of this book, tableware, contrast and its interaction with optimum lighting were discussed in detail in Chapter 4 along with a summary table of different tableware contrast designs. Briefly enhancing the colour contrast between plate, table and food in combination with optimum lighting levels and appropriate use of adapted tableware (including accessible tables for correct positioning at mealtimes) can help increase the amount of food consumed and improve eating abilities, therefore increasing independence (Prince et al., 2014).

Socialisation and stimulation

Mealtimes offer the greatest opportunity for socialisation and yet often they are looked upon as a task-focused caring duty (Batchelor-Murphy et al., 2015a). In a care home or group living setting people with dementia may be seated according to their current level of eating abilities. This may make mealtime tasks for carers easier to complete although it may be to the detriment of some of the individuals. Sitting someone with a friend or someone they have an affinity with provides a better environment for social interaction (Chaudhury et al., 2013). Eating must be a social occasion for people living with dementia. The focus of mealtime care needs to be more than just completing the 'task' of consuming food. As nicely described by one author, for the current generation of older people with dementia the ritual tradition of a family meal reinforced their role within the family and society. Food brought the family together, not just to eat but to provide support and share in each other's lives (Timlin and Rysenbry, 2010).

Mealtimes are a social experience; however for people with dementia in particular this experience can be either pleasant or unpleasant. Being in a 'noisy' or overstimulating dining room and being seated next to someone because of comparable levels of dependence instead of their social compatibility may contribute to a deterioration in eating abilities and meal behaviours. As dementia advances the person living with dementia can become increasingly socially isolated. Even within a care home, if someone's behaviour at mealtimes becomes worse, they disrupt others at mealtimes, their physical mobility declines or they simply find the mealtime stressful, they may choose or be encouraged to eat in their room. This increases isolation within their own place of living and may contribute to malnutrition and decreased quality of life. Eating is a social activity and support must be provided to encourage this for as long as possible. You often hear of care homes not having any financial budget for activities but rarely do you hear of the mealtime being used as a time for social activity. Ways to increase socialisation at mealtimes have been discussed in Chapter 6, and involved adapting the environment with changes to the serving styles of meals. This change to the style of food service may also improve the homelike feel of a mealtime, which is another environmental factor discussed later in this section.

Despite the importance of socialisation we should also remember that some people do like to eat alone. Perhaps they have been used to eating alone most of their life or just prefer to eat by themselves, or find the additional stimulation from having others present too much and feel overwhelmed. Eating with three or four others at a table may preserve independence in some, owing in part to socialisation and cuing from others, while some will show better independence eating with fewer people or on their own (Calkins, 2006). In a large, busy dining room, stimulation can be reduced by creating space and privacy using moveable dividers, a good example of which is provided in *Design for Dementia: Improving Dining and Bedroom Environments in Care Homes* (Timlin and Rysenbry, 2010, p.29). Importantly people with dementia have indicated that they require the choice to either have their own space to eat or have an area to talk to others (Chaudhury *et al.*, 2013). To increase socialisation in a care home it is important to consider seating arrangements. Sit the person with a friend or someone they have an affinity with to enhance social interaction, which may improve abilities. Or if already doing this, sit them with someone who has maintained eating abilities as this may help the individual continue to feed themselves by taking cues from others. This is preferred to sitting individuals based on comparable levels of dependence.

WALKING OR UNABLE TO SIT STILL AT MEALTIMES

Closely interrelated to socialisation and stimulation is the often-observed behaviour of 'wandering'. The term wandering was always used to describe someone with dementia walking throughout their residence. The issue with the word is that it tends to conjure up visions of someone aimlessly moving around without a purpose in an almost zombie-like fashion; the term walking is a far better description. Walking is a behavioural symptom of dementia and is unlikely to occur for no reason; it may be the person's response to unsupportive environmental influences, lack of stimulation or overstimulation, or other causes of discomfort or needs not being met. Walking is good for us or at the very least better than being sedentary, as long as it is not leading to increased energy needs which cannot be replaced by inadequate food intake. Walking should be supported for most people if it helps to preserve mobility and provides positive stimulation. It may have the added benefit of helping to prevent constipation or act as an appetite stimulant, for example. If the walking interrupts or prevents the person from engaging in a mealtime then suggestions for supporting this behaviour are provided in the following practical interventions chapter – Chapter 11. If an individual tends to walk or is impatient at mealtimes then it is important not to sit them in the dining room too long before food is served. You would not wait at the dinner table at home for 40 minutes before eating as you would likely get bored and want to leave. For a person with dementia, especially if the environment is unsupportive, this wait may cause an increase in agitation and loss of interest in food and lead to them walking away.

Carer interaction

As discussed in detail in the unsupportive environment section, the interaction between the carer and the person with dementia can affect meal behaviours and nutritional intake. What is not clear is what interactions help support meal behaviours and therefore decrease their occurrence (Gilmore-Bykovskyi, 2015). As dementia progresses, familiarity becomes more important and this also includes carers. People with later-stage dementia may not recognise a carer by name or maybe even face but may recognise their voice, touch, caring techniques and that they are there to help them. It is not uncommon for a person with dementia who requires feeding assistance to be more likely to accept food from a carer they have known for a period of time or they have some affinity with. The familiarity of a family member may be required to support someone to eat and may be appropriate for full feeding assistance or 'taking over' feeding when refusal is witnessed from carers. It has been shown that those individuals who have fewer family visits can have a higher risk of reduced food intake (Lin *et al.*, 2010). Person-centred interactions such as providing cueing techniques and offering choice have also been shown to be of benefit (Gilmore-Bykovskyi, 2015). Carers who provide assistance with feeding and who are personal, interested, involved, flexible, calm and cooperative achieve the best results (Smith and Greenwood, 2008).

Specific training techniques for dementia care such as the Montessori methods and spaced retrieval have also been shown to successfully support mealtime abilities and behaviours (W. Liu *et al.*, 2015). These types of training are very specific and usually out of the realm of the traditional carer and as such are not discussed in this book.

Homelike settings

It is difficult to define a 'one-size-fits-all' design of a dining room for people with dementia. The research on this subject suggests it should be themed on a small intimate homelike setting which helps to reduce noise and distractions while providing more social interaction opportunities (Chaudhury *et al.*, 2013). The non-institutional appearance of small dining rooms creates a more familiar mealtime environment and has been shown to reduce confusion (as to the function of the room) and improve food intake and eating abilities (Calkins, 2006). Adding recognisable objects as mentioned in Table 10.2 may help a person with dementia identify the mealtime setting and recall past memories and positive useful associations with food and mealtimes (Timlin and Rysenbry, 2010). Some research has indicated that people with dementia eating in care home dining rooms with more non-institutional features were less likely to have low food and fluid intakes (Reed *et al.*, 2005). Further research provides evidence that living in an unsupportive nursing home environment can lead to twice as many incidents of reduced mealtime abilities in people with dementia compared to those living in a supportive environment (Slaughter *et al.*, 2011).

Make sure the table settings are simple, as too many items or decorations can be distracting or confusing. If the décor articulates cultural preferences it may even help to promote a sense of belonging and ownership (Chaudhury *et al.*, 2013). In general, homelike dining rooms with simple paintings and plants, soft consistent lighting levels, tables set with high-contrast tablecloths/placemats/tableware and simple centrepieces along with appropriate music and sensory stimulation from the food itself would create a more familiar and appropriate environment in the dining room.

Determining the optimum number of people with dementia in the dining room in a care home setting is hard to define. One piece of research suggested that reducing numbers to 25–30 can increase food intake (Calkins, 2006) while smaller spaces with 5–12 people may provide optimum stimulation (Chaudhury et al., 2013). In a large care home rooms along a corridor leading to the main dining room could be turned into small dining areas to accommodate smaller dining spaces. Or the main dining area could be subdivided using dividers, low partitions and planters (Calkins, 2006).

Waiting for a long time before a meal or eating in an environment with many other people, thereby increasing sensory distraction and leading to confusion and agitation, are reasons for avoiding large communal dining areas. The intimate and more familiar ambience of a small dining room with non-institutional furniture and recognisable fixtures is associated with increased food intake and a reduction in meal behaviours (Prince et al., 2014). The distractions from excessive noise or stimulation are usually reduced through smaller dining arrangements.

Dining rooms that serve a dual or multiple purpose can trigger withdrawal and conflict between residents while carers can suffer from burnout. Keeping the dining room focused on food-related activities and not using it for non-food activities may help provide the familiarity needed for some to remember the room's purpose (Timlin and Rysenbry, 2010). If the dining room is also used for other activities then changing the layout and adding different tablecloths before mealtimes can help provide cues to some people with dementia that it is time for their next meal (Calkins, 2006). Additionally using wayfinding designs (such as signage that indicates the entrance to the room is the dining room, what time it is and what type of meal is being served) and large-print menus can provide orientation cues as to the purpose of the room (Brush et al., 2012). Using the aroma of certain foods, such as freshly baked bread or general cooking, could be used around mealtimes to orientate people to the mealtime and stimulate appetite (Chaudhury et al., 2013). Ideally each room in the living environment should have one activity associated with it thereby helping the person with dementia to maintain familiarity with the room's purpose (Timlin and Rysenbry, 2010).

Small, sturdy tables at the correct height

Both square and round tables have their own pros and cons. A square table sitting four people may be best for people with dementia as it helps define personal space but it can also enable socialisation, which is a key part of a mealtime experience (Chaudhury et al., 2013). Round tables on the other hand may be safer for people to move around as there are no sharp edges (Calkins, 2006). Perhaps what is more important is that the height of the table and chair allow the person full access to the table and that they can place their feet on the floor comfortably.

Style of food service

The style of food service and how this can improve socialisation and food intake was discussed in Chapter 6. Certain food service styles may also create a more homelike and familiar environment as well as providing social opportunities. Evidence indicates that being served at the table rather than pre-plated or on trays provides a more familiar dining environment and improved eating abilities and nutritional intake (Chaudhury et al., 2013). Certainly in a care home setting one would think that if everyone shared food at the table it would bring more of a sense of being at 'home'. The care home is after all where the residents live and this type of service allows a better sense of being involved in the mealtime experience. Compare this to a pre-plated meal which involves much less interaction and unfamiliarity. When was the last time someone served you a pre-made plate of food in your own home without you having any involvement?

It must be said however that if the pre-plated food involves food packaging then opening the packaging can become a factor affecting sufficient intake. This is commonly observed in both care homes and hospital settings (Weekes, 2008; Chaudhury et al., 2013; Walton et al., 2013). Avoiding using difficult-to-open food packaging may be all that is needed to improve eating abilities and nutrition in some individuals.

Studies have indicated that where people with dementia served their own food at the table, like a family-style food service, then they consumed more and engaged more (Charras and Frémontier, 2010). Previous research in older people living in care homes without dementia also found that 'family-style' mealtimes improved quality of life, physical performance and body weight over a six-month time period when compared to typical pre-plated service style (Nijs et al.,

2006). This type of service may not work practically in care homes for every meal but these can always be adapted and certainly may be worth considering for foods all served from one main dish, for example shepherd's pie or lasagne. Without this active participation by people with dementia too often mealtimes are under the complete control of carers (Hung *et al.*, 2016), which may be a negative factor to nutritional intake for many. Table 10.3 describes the three most common meal service styles typically used, how these serving styles may impact on familiarity and at what stage of dementia they may be better indicated for use.

Table 10.3: Meal service styles to improve familiarity and homelike appearance

Serving style	How it works	Potential benefits
Restaurant	Meals are chosen via a menu and are provided in a pre-plated form	Provides little social interaction and may be best suited to those with mild dementia
Buffet	Meals are provided in a bulk service style where carers show the food available to choose from	Provides more social interaction between carer and person with dementia Increases the use of sense through visually seeing the food and smelling the food aromas Can help with appropriate choice of food and portion sizes May be more beneficial for those with moderate to severe dementia
Family	Meals are provided at the table with everyone sharing from the same dish	Increases social interaction between carers and persons with dementia, and among the persons with dementia May provide the most familiar serving style to those with severe dementia Increases the use of the senses and food choice as mentioned above

The effect of environmental change on staff

When discussing the evidence around manipulating the mealtime environment to better support people with dementia there is an important factor which has occurred during the research into this topic. This very interesting but unverified factor is the effect that environmental changes may have on the carer.

One piece of research which used a case study approach in a dementia care home utilised improved lighting (optimised to those with dementia) and modified tableware (colour contrast) as an effective intervention. The residents with 'mid-stage' Alzheimer's disease who participated in the study increased their calorie and fluid intake and increased their functional independence and social engagement at mealtimes (Brush et al., 2002). In other words they were able to eat more independently as their eating abilities were better supported; they increased their nutritional intake; plus they engaged with staff and other residents more. Intriguingly the authors found the changes affected staff positivity as well (Brush, 2001; Brush et al., 2002). Carers commented: 'it is nicer to work here' and 'more cheery in the dining room'. The environmental changes also aided in helping engage staff with residents. For example, making new table settings increased social interaction between staff and residents. Changing the environment, it seems, could be an untapped source of motivation and improved job satisfaction for carers while enabling them both to be more attentive and provide better care at mealtimes. Therefore apart from the actual environmental interventions put in place (enhanced lighting and modified tableware), the increased social interaction and improved carer attentiveness may be the reasons for an improvement in outcomes (increased food intake and eating abilities). Interestingly enough about halfway through this real-life case-study research project there was a change in staffing policy leading to one more member of staff being available at mealtimes to provide assistance. This most likely affected outcomes as well although it would have been impossible to measure accurately. More staff probably meant more interactions and improved attentiveness with the residents, which may have led to the improved eating abilities and independence. Nevertheless we can assume the changes to the environment along with additional staff and happier carers all meant better quality of life for those being cared for. It is important to remember this as many interventions put in place are solely reliable on the staff to initiate them, monitor them and adapt them to the person. Changing the environment obviously does not increase staff numbers but certainly may provide happier staff and a better environment for carers to perform their caring roles.

Supplementary to the case study just mentioned, many environmental modifications to both the dining room and care home were made in another interesting dementia care home study (Mamhidir *et al.*, 2007). Changes included making mealtime settings more 'homelike' and adapting the dining equipment and the type of service by introducing a 'self-service' into bowls at the table rather than the usual service style of pre-prepared trays. Staff reported that this self-service style and other environmental changes helped to increase contact between residents, and the mealtime atmosphere was more pleasant. In addition to environmental changes, training on improved communication techniques such as using cueing techniques (as discussed in Chapter 4) and empathy were provided to carers before the environmental changes were made. All of these changes helped the care staff become more attentive to each person's needs. This may have been the main factor in improving outcomes of increased weight in 13 out of 18 residents. In comparison only 2 out of 15 residents increased weight in the non-randomised control group. A very high risk of recruitment and intervention bias limits the generalisation of this study; however, it shows that if a supportive mealtime environment and appropriate carer support are provided, increased nutrition and body weight can be achieved. This type of research bias does not matter in the real-life setting of course. Simply modifying the mealtime environment while providing training helped the staff provide better care at mealtimes and in the carers' own words made a more 'pleasant atmosphere'. The use of self-service – all serve and eat from one source – is a novel idea and one perhaps some care homes and people in their own homes could adopt. The self-service seemed to increase social interaction just as the mealtime environmental changes did in the previous case study mentioned (Brush *et al.*, 2002). Therefore to enhance socialisation for people with dementia these simple modifications should be tried and monitored for effectiveness.

Little is really known about how a more supportive mealtime environment impacts on carers' practices or what specific changes in the environment enable them to provide more effective care (Hung *et al.*, 2016). Perhaps a supportive mealtime environment allows opportunities for carers and those they care for to better interact – socially increasing the wellbeing of the person with dementia and the job satisfaction of the carer.

Summary

Despite esteemed researchers identifying the benefits of supportive mealtime environments almost two decades ago this information has not managed to penetrate all care settings. There has also been a lack of repeat research investigations into these initial findings and as such the quality of the research is not strong, making it hard to prove a significant benefit for improving meal behaviours (Whear *et al.*, 2014).

Research conducted mainly in care homes indicates that a supportive mealtime environment and training focused on mealtime care in those with later-stage dementia can achieve increased calorie intake (Prince *et al.*, 2014). The mealtime environment can be easily modified to compensate for reduced mealtime abilities, while an unsupportive environment seems to exert a negative influence on people with dementia. Creating a supportive mealtime environment may have particular positive effects on meal behaviours. Supportive mealtime modifications include small dining rooms, homelike atmosphere, appropriate lighting and colour contrast, minimised noise, music, orientation cues and furniture grouping to foster social interactions (Chaudhury *et al.*, 2013). Insufficient evidence exists to make any clear recommendations regarding the content of the mealtime environment but a flexible, individualised and person-centred care approach in settings that resemble homes is suggested (Prince *et al.*, 2014).

Surely one of the most interesting findings from research into the mealtime environment is the impact on care staff. By creating a supportive mealtime environment it seems to allow staff more time or availability to hone in on individuals' needs and achieve more effective interactions. This is extremely interesting as it has been reported that there can be a complete lack of interaction between carers and people with dementia, with as little as two minutes' interaction for every hour (Timlin and Rysenbry, 2010). Therefore interaction at mealtimes, which are supposed to be a social occasion, can benefit from improved environment and are important for the wellbeing of the person with dementia and the job satisfaction of the carer. A change in the environment has been linked with a change in staff culture, helping them to become more person centred (Chaudhury *et al.*, 2013).

Re-decorating a building or buying new 'dementia-friendly' tableware can be costly, not to mention disruptive, and as the research shows that this will not guarantee it will work for everyone, it wastes valuable resources. A lack of quality in the research of interventions means their effectiveness is not fully known and may be detrimental as well as beneficial; therefore assessment and monitoring are extremely important. A person-centred approach is to be adopted by assessing and monitoring each individual so interventions can be tailored to that individual's needs. This is especially true in care homes where interventions impact the group; for example, a complete change to the colour of all the plates may negatively affect many residents living there.

The fourth section of the DMAT can help identify problems with the environment if a person experiences the meal behaviours highlighted in this chapter. Specific environmental assessment tools can also be used to look more widely at the dining and other living environments, as discussed earlier.

11

Practical Interventions Section 4

SUPPORTING MEAL BEHAVIOURS THROUGH ADJUSTING THE MEALTIME ENVIRONMENT

Assessment

Table 11.1 shows section 4 of the Dementia Mealtime Assessment Tool (DMAT, 2017) as described in Chapter 3. This section focuses on assessing the meal behaviours often observed in people with later-stage dementia. Assess the meal behaviour of the person so that appropriate changes to the environment and care practices can be introduced or improved.

Table 11.1: The DMAT section 4: Assessment of meal behaviours

Mealtime observations: Meal behaviours	Please tick observed abilities		
	Not seen	Seen once	Seen repeatedly
1. Hoards, hides, throws or plays with food			
2. Eats other people's food (or drink)			
3. Refuses to eat (verbally or physically)			
4. Bats away or pushes away spoon presented by carer			
5. Turns head away when being fed			
6. Distracted from eating			
7. Demonstrates impatient behaviour around mealtimes			
8. Eats small amounts and leaves table			
9. Walks during mealtime or unable to sit still for meals			
10. Shows agitated behaviour or irritability			

Interventions

It is much harder to have specific interventions for meal behaviours compared to reduced eating abilities or oral abilities. Many factors make up the environment and it can be hard to precisely know what environmental change will have the most impact. Multiple interventions used at the same time may provide the most effective option for improving a range of health outcomes.

Implementing interventions is never simple and the carer(s) will need to adopt a trial-and-error approach ensuring that both successes and failures are documented on a care plan. Carers need to be aware that interventions can potentially worsen meal behaviours or eating abilities. Monitoring the effectiveness of chosen interventions regularly, for example every two to four weeks, is key to defining the right intervention at the right time for the right person. One of the main difficulties in group living facilities such as care homes is modifying the environment to support all the needs of all the residents. By assessing and monitoring each individual, carers can help create a person-centred approach ensuring the interventions are directed to supporting the individual's current level of cognitive and physical functioning.

Guidance for interventions

- Many of the common meal behaviours identified in the DMAT will fall into similar themes: agitation, impatience and resisting care. The interventions used to support these behaviours often overlap and therefore some meal behaviours will require the use of the same interventions.

- As described throughout the book, interventions follow a hierarchy of suggestions from simple to more complex. Therefore in regards to the mealtime environment this starts with simple cueing techniques, followed by modifications to table settings or tableware. Additional adjustments to the mealtime environment can improve noise levels, under- or over-stimulation and create a familiar environment. Further interventions are aimed at enhanced socialisation through changing food service styles, seating and table arrangements, or if required, providing full feeding assistance.

- In combination with environmental changes both adapting the food and texture of the food may be indicated, as can a referral to appropriate healthcare professionals.

- When considering individual preferences, such as food likes and dislikes and mealtime eating patterns, discuss with the resident first along with any family or friends.

- CARE HOME SPECIFIC: The vast majority of suggested interventions can be applied to different settings, for example home care, care home, acute care, independent living and so on. However the majority of research has been conducted in care home/long-term care settings and some interventions will only be applicable to these settings and will be labelled 'CARE HOME SPECIFIC'.

- IMPORTANT NOTICE: Some reduced abilities can indicate further assessment may be required or that the patient may be at increased risk at mealtimes. If this is the case for the list of interventions available to enhance this reduced ability an 'IMPORTANT NOTICE' will be highlighted at the start of the intervention list. It is important to read and understand what this means in relation to the person who is being cared for and act appropriately to prevent any harm to the person.

Suggested interventions for adjusting the mealtime environment to support meal behaviours

1. Hoards, hides, throws or plays with food

- Modify table setting:

   - Keep other people's food out of reach. Remove non-food items from the table to help define each person's eating area. Keep food-related items to a minimum on the table.

- Increase socialisation:

   - Find outlets for the person's energy: they may be looking for something to do. Involve them in activities. Give the person a role in meal service, for example setting table, pouring water and helping others to the table. Alternatively try using art, music or other activities to help engage the person and divert attention away from the meal behaviour.

- Provide cueing:

  - Try serving small amounts of food at a time and monitor intake.

  - Try verbal cues and verbal prompting to encourage the person to eat, and explain what they are eating using positive descriptors.

  - Remove the meal for five to ten minutes, then serve again and offer encouragement.

- Adjust environment:

  - Introduce relaxing music to suit the person's preferences as this can improve meal behaviours. Be aware of unsupportive environmental influences and adjust as required, for example inappropriate lighting levels affecting vision, auditory distractions secondary to overstimulating noise levels, inappropriate tableware with poor colour contrast, an institutional appearance that doesn't represent a familiar homelike environment, overstimulation or understimulation at the meal setting and lack of socialisation.

- Full assistance:

  - If all suggestions fail then consider the need for full supervision at mealtimes especially if food intake is reduced and weight is lost.

- CARE HOME SPECIFIC: Increase socialisation:

  - Consider seating arrangements. Sit the person with a friend or someone they have an affinity with to enhance social interaction, which may improve the behaviour. Or if already doing this sit them with someone who has maintained mealtime abilities as this may help them by taking cues from others (rather than seating based on assistance needs).

2. Eats other people's food (or drink)

- IMPORTANT NOTICE: If the person has dysphagia (swallowing difficulty) then problems with the social environment at mealtimes including eating food not appropriate for the person may be a risk factor for a negative health consequence (asphyxiation and/or choking episode, aspiration incidents, dehydration and poor nutritional status)

- Modify table setting:

  - Keep other people's food out of reach. Remove non-food items from the table to help define each person's eating area. Keep food-related items to a minimum on the table.

  - Sit the person on a square table rather than round table as this may help identify boundaries. Square tables create a sense of 'my space'; round tables can create the illusion of someone eating off another's plate.

- Modify tableware:

  - Trial visual cueing for boundaries by using large visual place mats to reduce interest in another's meal.

- Provide cueing:

  - Try labelling the meal setting with the person's name or even name the items of food if possible. For example wrap a sandwich and label it, then help unwrap if required.

  - Sit nearby and verbally encourage the person to eat from their own plate, and remind them what they are eating and where their own food and boundaries are.

- Adjust environment:

  - Be aware of unsupportive environmental influences and adjust as required, for example inappropriate lighting levels affecting vision, auditory distractions secondary to overstimulating noise levels, inappropriate tableware with poor colour contrast, an institutional appearance that doesn't represent a familiar homelike environment, overstimulation or understimulation at the meal setting and lack of socialisation.

- Modify serving style:

   - Trial serving small amounts of food at a time or serve in courses, quickly replacing the food as it is consumed.

- Increase socialisation:

   - Adapting the service style may improve the meal behaviour. For example provide the opportunity for the person to serve their own food or share food from the same large dish (family style) or show the food before serving it (buffet style) rather than serving pre-plated food. This can also improve portion size chosen and provide increased food choice.

   - Try eating your meal with the person. Eating with company can enhance mealtime abilities owing to social interaction and taking cues to eat from others. In addition you can help keep their focus on the meal and provide appropriate assistance if required to help maintain food intake. It can also help carers become more aware of individual likes, dislikes and preferences.

- Full assistance:

   - If all suggestions fail then consider the need for full supervision at mealtimes.

- CARE HOME SPECIFIC: Increase socialisation:

   - Consider seating arrangements. Sit the person with a friend or someone they have an affinity with to enhance social interaction, which may improve the behaviour. Or if already doing this sit them with someone who has maintained mealtime abilities as this may help them by taking cues from others (rather than seating based on assistance needs).

   - If the meal behaviour is affecting other people's food intake then consider sitting the person on a single table and, once others have finished eating move the person to sit with them.

3. Refuses to eat (verbally or physically)

- IMPORTANT NOTICE: Food may be refused due to an underlying physical problem, such as a swallowing difficulty. If you suspect this please liaise with a speech and language pathologist/therapist (SLP/SLT) immediately for advice. Do not argue. This usually leads to confrontation and escalation of the meal behaviour. Do not attempt to force-feed the person. Following a range of interventions to prompt them to eat, if they still refuse then stop the meal to prevent distressing them and try again at the next snack or mealtime.

- Provide cueing:

  - Remove the meal for five to ten minutes, then serve again and offer encouragement.

  - Try verbal cues and verbal prompting to encourage the person to eat, and explain what they are eating using a positive description.

  - Check food preferences. The person may not like the food any more. To evaluate possible solutions, record specific behaviours such as moods, foods accepted and refused, successful strategies and times of day the food is presented. Ensure food preferences are recorded and ask the person, family or friends for information on food habits and preferences. The use of life story work can aid this process.

  - Try a more expressive act such as gently touching the forearm or gently rubbing the top of the person's hand to get their attention and then focus them on the meal.

  - If the person requires feeding assistance then consider humming songs while assisting as this may improve the meal behaviour.

- Adjust environment:

  - Introduce relaxing music to suit the person's preferences as this can improve meal behaviours. Be aware of unsupportive environmental influences and adjust as required, for example, inappropriate lighting levels affecting vision, auditory distractions secondary to overstimulating noise levels, inappropriate tableware with poor colour contrast, an institutional appearance that doesn't represent a familiar homelike environment, overstimulation or understimulation at the meal setting and lack of socialisation.

  - If possible move the person to a less distracting environment and continue feeding, or provide support with the mealtime. For example try providing meals in a smaller, more intimate room with fewer people, or use room dividers to create this effect to reduce overstimulation.

- Adapt food:

  - Ensure other choices of food and drink are available at mealtimes to replace the refused food, including foods the individual favours.

  - Trial finger foods which may be better accepted and allow more independence with self-feeding.

  - If food intake is often difficult but drinks are consumed more easily then try offering more nourishing drinks to replace the missed food.

- Increase socialisation:

  - Adapting the service style may improve the meal behaviour. For example provide the opportunity for the person to serve their own food or share food from the same large dish (family style) or show the food before serving it (buffet style) rather than serving pre-plated food. This can also improve portion size chosen and provide increased food choice.

  - Try eating your meal with the person. Eating with company can enhance mealtime abilities owing to social interaction and taking cues to eat from others. In addition you can help keep their focus on the meal and provide appropriate assistance if required to help maintain food intake. It can also help carers become more aware of individuals' likes, dislikes and preferences.

- Eating together (family style) on small round tables, increasing social interaction through welcoming individuals to the dining room or using an informal activity before eating, for example flower arranging, may prompt better attention and meal behaviours.

- Texture modification:

  - Trial a different food texture by providing softer foods that are easier to chew and swallow. Use the Dysphagia Diet Food Texture Descriptors or IDDSI Framework and Descriptors to define the correct soft consistency if a swallowing difficulty has been identified.

- Modify tableware:

  - If the carer is currently providing feeding assistance then reassess this need and encourage self-feeding if possible. Trial using adapted cutlery and crockey such as a scoop plate and spoon, and provide cueing and encouragement.

- Enhance familiarity:

  - The person may benefit from receiving assistance from one specific carer or have consistency in feeding assistance or mealtime practices. With advancing dementia people need to recognise their carers or somehow realise they are there to assist with eating.

  - Ask if a family member can help to support or feed the person, especially if they have assisted at mealtimes previously, as this may provide more familiarity.

  - Try to prepare familiar foods in familiar ways, especially foods that are favourites or culturally significant, to help with food recognition.

- CARE HOME SPECIFIC: Increase socialisation:

  - Consider seating arrangements. Sit the person with a friend or someone they have an affinity with to enhance social interaction, which may improve the behaviour. Or if already doing this sit them with someone who has maintained mealtime abilities as this may help them by taking cues from others (rather than seating based on assistance needs).

- REFERRAL: A medication review may be appropriate. Certain drugs can have side effects that impact on eating and drinking, for example causing nausea or constipation. Consult with the individual's doctor. If the meal behaviour persists and dietary intake is reduced and weight is lost refer to a dietitian for nutritional assessment.

4. Bats away or pushes away spoon presented by carer

The interventions to be implemented to support this meal behaviour are the same as number 3, 'Refuses to eat (verbally or physically)'. Continue to pay attention to the 'important notice' and 'referral' [to health professionals] as indicated.

- IMPORTANT NOTICE: Do not attempt to force-feed the person. Following a range of interventions to prompt them to eat, if they still refuse then stop the meal to prevent distressing them and try again at the next snack or mealtime.

- REFERRAL: If the meal behaviour persists, dietary intake is reduced and weight is lost, refer to a dietitian for nutritional assessment.

5. Turns their head away when being fed

The interventions to be implemented to support this meal behaviour are the same as number 3, 'Refuses to eat (verbally or physically)'. Continue to pay attention to the 'important notice' and 'referral' [to health professionals] as indicated.

- IMPORTANT NOTICE: Do not attempt to force-feed the person. Following a range of interventions to prompt them to eat, if they still refuse then stop the meal to prevent distressing them and try again at the next snack or mealtime.

- REFERRAL: If the meal behaviour persists, dietary intake is reduced and weight is lost, refer to a dietitian for nutritional assessment.

6. Distracted from eating

- IMPORTANT NOTICE: If the person has dysphagia (swallowing difficulty) then distractibility at mealtimes is a medium-risk factor for a negative health consequence (asphyxiation and/or choking episode, aspiration incidents, dehydration and poor nutritional status) (Joliffe and Chadwick, 2006).

- Provide cueing:

    - Make sure the person is not alerted to meals too early and is not sitting for a long period of time with nothing to do before the meal is served.

    - Use verbal cues and verbal prompting to keep the person's attention directed to the mealtime; for example show them and tell them what is on their plate and frequently remind them what they are doing.

    - Use manual prompts to gently assist the person with eating; for example place cutlery back in their hands, and guide their focus back to the meal.

    - Try a more expressive act such as gently touching the forearm or gently rubbing the top of the person's hand to get their attention and then focus them on the meal.

    - Try modelling eating so the person can copy your movements and offer encouragement.

- Adjust environment:

    - Make sure the room is calm and quiet, that the person has everything needed for the meal (for example their glasses/dentures/hearing aid), has been to the toilet and is sitting comfortably.

- – Reduce competing sensory stimulation to focus the person's attention on eating; for example turn off the TV and stop other non-meal activities or unnecessary noise. If possible prevent people from entering and leaving the room or use dividers to separate the walkway from tables.

- – Introduce relaxing music to suit the person's preferences as this can improve meal behaviours. Be aware of unsupportive environmental influences and adjust as required, for example inappropriate lighting levels affecting vision, auditory distractions secondary to overstimulating noise levels, inappropriate tableware with poor colour contrast, an institutional appearance that doesn't represent a familiar homelike environment, overstimulation or understimulation at the meal setting and lack of socialisation.

- – If possible move the person to a less distracting environment and continue feeding or provide support with the mealtime. For example try providing meals in a smaller, more intimate room with fewer people, or use room dividers to create this effect to reduce overstimulation.

- – If someone who is more confused/agitated is positioned next to a noisy or distracting environment (e.g. a corridor or doorway) then move them to a more appropriate position to reduce excess environmental stimulation.

- Modify table setting:

  - – Remove non-food items and keep food-related items to a minimum on the table.

  - – Simplify the meal process by placing only one plate and one utensil on the table, directly in front of the person. Only serve one course at a time so that the necessity of making choices is limited and there are fewer distractions. *Note*: when using only one plate and a spoon the use of a scoop plate may be required.

  - – Sometimes a crowded plate is overstimulating for those who are easily distracted and overwhelmed. Try providing one plate with one food at a time. When the person is finished with the first dish, replace it with another.

- Increase socialisation:

  - Adapting the service style may improve the meal behaviour. For example provide the opportunity for the person to serve their own food or share food from the same large dish (family style) or show the food before serving it (buffet style) rather than being serving pre-plated food. This can also improve portion size chosen and provide increased food choice.

  - Try eating your meal with the person. Eating with company can enhance mealtime abilities owing to social interaction and taking cues to eat from others. In addition you can help keep their focus on the meal and provide appropriate assistance if required to help maintain food intake. It can also help carers become more aware of individuals' likes, dislikes and preferences.

  - Eating together (family style) on small round tables, increasing social interaction through welcoming individuals to the dining room, or using an informal activity before eating, for example flower arranging, may prompt better attention and meal behaviours.

- Modify serving style:

  - Consider whether the person would prefer to eat by themselves. Not everyone likes to eat with others and they may find the stimulation from others overwhelming. Trial serving on a single table and monitor intake.

- Enhance familiarity:

  - Minimise any institutional appearance by removing equipment or unnecessary items when not in use to avoid overstimulation, and make the meal setting look like a traditional 'homelike' mealtime.

- CARE HOME SPECIFIC: Increase socialisation:

  - Consider seating arrangements. Sit the person with a friend or someone they have an affinity with to enhance social interaction, which may improve the behaviour. Or if already doing this sit them with someone who has maintained mealtime abilities as this may help them by taking cues from others (rather than seating based on assistance needs).

- REFERRAL: If the meal behaviour persists, dietary intake is reduced and weight is lost, refer to a dietitian for nutritional assessment.

7. Demonstrates impatient behaviour around mealtimes

- Provide cueing:

  - Make sure the person is not alerted to meals too early and is not sitting for a long period of time with nothing to do before the meal is served.

- Adjust environment:

  - Make sure the room is calm and quiet, that the person has everything needed for the meal (for example their glasses/dentures/hearing aid), has been to the toilet and is sitting comfortably.

  - Introduce relaxing music to suit the person's preferences as this can improve meal behaviours. Be aware of unsupportive environmental influences and adjust as required, for example inappropriate lighting levels affecting vision, auditory distractions secondary to overstimulating noise levels, inappropriate tableware with poor colour contrast, an institutional appearance that doesn't represent a familiar homelike environment, overstimulation or understimulation at the meal setting and lack of socialisation.

- Modify serving style:

  - Serve the person their meal before other people and/or minimise waiting times for this person if offering food in courses.

- Increase socialisation:

  - Find outlets for the person's energy; they may be looking for something to do. Involve them in activities. Give the person a role in meal service, for example setting table, pouring water and helping others to the table.

- Adapt food:

  - If appetite is normally good and the meal intake will not be reduced, offer something to eat while they wait for the meal to arrive, for example some simple canapés.

- Enhance familiarity:

  - Respect routines around food and drink at mealtimes. Try to discover if the person has habits that have been disrupted and change the routine to make it as familiar as possible. The use of life story work can help aid this process.

- Increase socialisation:

  - Adapting the service style may improve the meal behaviour. For example provide the opportunity for the person to serve their own food or share food from the same large dish (family style) or show the food before serving it (buffet style) rather than serving pre-plated food. This can also improve portion size chosen and provide increased food choice.

  - Try eating your meal with the person. Eating with company can enhance mealtime abilities owing to social interaction and taking cues to eat from others. In addition you can help keep their focus on the meal and provide appropriate assistance if required to help maintain food intake. It can also help carers become more aware of individuals' likes, dislikes and preferences.

  - Eating together (family style) on small round tables, increasing social interaction through welcoming individuals to the dining room or using an informal activity before eating, for example flower arranging, may prompt better attention and meal behaviours.

- Food First advice:
    - If there is a time of day when the person is less impatient (e.g. morning/breakfast time) ensure a good variety of food is on offer at this time to maximise intake.

- CARE HOME SPECIFIC: Increase socialisation:
    - Consider seating arrangements. Sit the person with a friend or someone they have an affinity with to enhance social interaction, which may improve the behaviour. Or if already doing this sit them with someone who has maintained mealtime abilities as this may help them by taking cues from others (rather than seating based on assistance needs).

- REFERRAL: If the meal behaviour persists, dietary intake is reduced and weight is lost, refer to a dietitian for nutritional assessment.

8. Eats small amounts and leaves table

- IMPORTANT NOTICE: If the person has dysphagia (swallowing difficulty) then behavioural difficulties at mealtimes are a medium-risk factor for a negative health consequence (asphyxiation and/or choking episode, aspiration incidents, dehydration and poor nutritional status) (Joliffe and Chadwick, 2006).

- Provide cueing:
    - Make sure the person is not alerted to meals too early and is not sitting for a long period of time with nothing to do before the meal is served.
    - Use verbal cues and verbal prompting to keep the person's attention directed to the mealtime; for example show them and tell them what is on their plate and frequently remind them what they are doing.

- Adjust environment:
    - Make sure the room is calm and quiet, that the person has everything needed for the meal (for example their glasses/

dentures/hearing aid), has been to the toilet and is sitting comfortably.

– Reduce competing sensory stimulation to focus the person's attention on eating; for example turn off the TV and stop other non-meal activities or unnecessary noise. If possible prevent people from entering and leaving the room or use dividers to separate walkways from tables.

– Introduce relaxing music to suit the person's preferences as this can improve meal behaviours. Be aware of unsupportive environmental influences and adjust as required, for example inappropriate lighting levels affecting vision, auditory distractions secondary to overstimulating noise levels, inappropriate tableware with poor colour contrast, an institutional appearance that doesn't represent a familiar homelike environment, overstimulation or understimulation at the meal setting and lack of socialisation.

– 'Camouflage' doors to reduce 'exit-seeking behaviour', or sit the person with their back to the door so they are less inclined to leave.

– If possible move the person to a less distracting environment and continue feeding or provide support with the mealtime. For example try providing meals in a smaller, more intimate room with fewer people, or use room dividers to create this effect to reduce overstimulation.

– The use of calming music can help create a relaxing atmosphere and may reduce agitation (especially verbal and physically non-aggressive behaviours) or irritability.

• Enhance familiarity:

– Respect routines around food and drink at mealtimes. Try to discover if the person has habits that have been disrupted, and change the routine to make it as familiar as possible. The use of life story work can help with this process.

- Food First advice:

  - If there is a time of day when the person is less impatient (e.g. morning/breakfast time) ensure a good variety of food is on offer at this time to maximise intake.

  - Provide visible snacks in the lounges and rooms that the person frequents so they can help themselves. Also offer encouragement.

  - Try limiting the number of foods available at any one time and instead provide little and often, focusing on protein and energy (calorie) dense sources first.

  - Provide small frequent meals; for example five or six meals per day may be needed for individuals who are unable to eat much at any one time.

- Increase socialisation:

  - Adapting the service style may improve the meal behaviour. For example provide the opportunity for the person to serve their own food or share food from the same large dish (family style) or show the food before serving it (buffet style) rather than serving pre-plated food. This can also improve portion size chosen and provide increased food choice.

  - Try eating your meal with the person. Eating with company can enhance mealtime abilities owing to social interaction and taking cues to eat from others. In addition you can help keep their focus on the meal and provide appropriate assistance if required to help maintain food intake. It can also help carers become more aware of individuals' likes, dislikes and preferences.

  - Eating together (family style) on small round tables, increasing social interaction through welcoming individuals to the dining room or using an informal activity before eating (for example flower arranging) may prompt better attention and meal behaviours.

- Adapt food:

  - To continue eating, encourage the use of finger food to take away from the mealtime or have while walking (you could provide a pouch if acceptable).

- Adapt drinks:

  - Carry drinks in cartons or use bottles as they are easier to carry around.

- CARE HOME SPECIFIC: Increase socialisation:

  - Consider seating arrangements. Sit the person with a friend or someone they have an affinity with to enhance social interaction, which may improve the behaviour. Or if already doing this sit them with someone who has maintained mealtime abilities as this may help them by taking cues from others (rather than seating based on assistance needs).

- REFERRAL: If the meal behaviour persists, dietary intake is reduced and weight is lost, refer to a dietitian for nutritional assessment.

9. Walks during mealtime or unable to sit still for meals

- Adjust environment:

  - The use of calming music can help create a relaxing atmosphere and may reduce agitation (especially verbal and physically non-aggressive behaviours) or irritability.

  - Make sure the room is calm and quiet, that the person has everything needed for the meal (for example their glasses/dentures/hearing aid), has been to the toilet and is sitting comfortably.

  - Reduce competing sensory stimulation to focus the person's attention on eating; for example turn off the TV and stop other non-meal activities or unnecessary noise. If possible prevent people from entering and leaving the room or use dividers to separate walkways from tables.

- – Introduce relaxing music to suit the person's preferences as this can improve meal behaviours. Be aware of unsupportive environmental influences and adjust as required, for example inappropriate lighting levels affecting vision, auditory distractions secondary to overstimulating noise levels, inappropriate tableware with poor colour contrast, an institutional appearance that doesn't represent a familiar homelike environment, overstimulation or understimulation at the meal setting and lack of socialisation.

- – 'Camouflage' doors to reduce 'exit-seeking behaviour'. Or sit the person with their back to the door so they are less inclined to leave.

- – If possible move the person to a less distracting environment and continue feeding or provide support with the mealtime. For example try providing meals in a smaller, more intimate room with fewer people. Or use room dividers to create this effect to reduce overstimulation.

- • Provide cueing:

- – Use verbal cues and verbal prompting to keep the person's attention directed to the mealtime; for example show them and tell them what is on their plate and frequently remind them what they are doing.

- – Make sure the person is not alerted to meals too early and is not sitting for a long period of time with nothing to do before the meal is served.

- – Use manual prompts to gently guide the person back to the table or place cutlery back in their hands.

- • Increase socialisation:

- – Walk with the person before a meal and plan a route that ends with a mealtime where you sit together.

- • Enhance familiarity:

- – Respect routines around food and drink at mealtimes. Try to discover if the person has habits that have been disrupted, and change the routine to make it as familiar as possible. The use of life story work can help aid this process.

- Food First advice:

  - If there is a time of day when the person is less impatient (e.g. morning/breakfast time) ensure a good variety of food is on offer at this time to maximise intake.

  - Provide visible snacks in the lounges and rooms that the person frequents so they can help themselves. Also offer encouragement.

  - Try limiting the number of foods available at any one time and instead provide little and often, focusing on protein and energy (calorie) dense sources first.

- Increase socialisation:

  - Adapting the service style may improve the meal behaviour. For example provide the opportunity for the person to serve their own food or share food from the same large dish (family style) or show the food before serving it (buffet style) rather than serving pre-plated food. This can also improve portion size chosen and provide increased food choice.

  - Try eating your meal with the person. Eating with company can enhance mealtime abilities owing to social interaction and taking cues to eat from others. In addition you can help keep their focus on the meal and provide appropriate assistance if required to help maintain food intake. It can also help carers become more aware of individuals' likes, dislikes and preferences.

  - Eating together (family style) on small round tables, increasing social interaction through welcoming individuals to the dining room or using an informal activity before eating (for example flower arranging) may prompt better attention and meal behaviours.

- Adapt food:

  - To continue eating, encourage the use of finger food to take away from the mealtime or to have while walking (you could provide a pouch if acceptable).

- Adapt drinks:

  - Carry drinks in cartons or use bottles as they are easier to carry around.

- CARE HOME SPECIFIC: Increase socialisation:

  - Consider seating arrangements. Sit the person with a friend or someone they have an affinity with to enhance social interaction, which may improve the behaviour. Or if already doing this sit them with someone who has maintained mealtime abilities as this may help them by taking cues from others (rather than seating based on assistance needs).

- REFERRAL: If the meal behaviour persists, dietary intake is reduced and weight is lost, refer to a dietitian for nutritional assessment.

10. Shows agitated behaviour or irritability

- IMPORTANT NOTICE: If the person has dysphagia (swallowing difficulty) then behavioural difficulties at mealtimes are a high-risk factor for a negative health consequence (asphyxiation and/or choking episode, aspiration incidents, dehydration and poor nutritional status) (Joliffe and Chadwick, 2006).

- Provide cueing:

  - Make sure the person is not alerted to meals too early and is not sitting for a long period of time with nothing to do before the meal is served.

  - Reassure and remind the person where they are and what they are doing.

- Adjust environment:
  - Make sure the room is calm and quiet, that the person has everything needed for the meal (for example their glasses/dentures/hearing aid), has been to the toilet and is sitting comfortably.

  - Reduce competing sensory stimulation to focus the person's attention on eating; for example turn off the TV and stop other non-meal activities or unnecessary noise. If possible prevent people from entering and leaving the room or use dividers to separate walkways from tables.

  - Be aware of unsupportive environmental influences and adjust as required, for example inappropriate lighting levels affecting vision, auditory distractions secondary to overstimulating noise levels, inappropriate tableware with poor colour contrast, an institutional appearance that doesn't represent a familiar homelike environment, overstimulation or understimulation at the meal setting and lack of socialisation.

  - The use of calming music can help create a relaxing atmosphere and may reduce agitation (especially verbal and physically non-aggressive behaviours) or irritability.

  - If someone who is more confused/agitated is positioned next to a noisy or distracting environment (e.g. a corridor or doorway) then move them to a more appropriate position to reduce excess environmental stimulation.

  - If possible move the person to a less distracting environment and continue feeding or provide support with the mealtime. For example try providing meals in a smaller, more intimate room with fewer people. Or use room dividers to create this effect to reduce overstimulation.

- Modify serving style:
  - Serve the person their meal before other people and/or minimise waiting times for them if offering food in courses.

- If the person requires feeding assistance then consider humming songs while assisting as this may improve the meal behaviour.

- Enhance familiarity:

  - Minimise any institutional appearance by removing equipment or unnecessary items when not in use to avoid overstimulation, and make the meal setting look like a traditional 'homelike' mealtime.

  - The person may benefit from receiving assistance from one specific carer or having consistency in feeding or mealtime practices. With advancing dementia people need to recognise their carers or somehow realise they are there to assist with eating.

- Increase socialisation:

  - Find outlets for the person's energy. They may be looking for something to do; involve them in activities. Give the person a role in meal service, for example setting table, pouring water and helping others to the table. Alternatively try using art, music or other activities to help engage the person and divert attention away from the anxiety.

  - Adapting the service style may improve the meal behaviour. For example provide the opportunity for the person to serve their own food or share food from the same large dish (family style) or show the food before serving it (buffet style) rather than serving pre-plated food. This can also improve portion size chosen and provide increased food choice.

  - Try eating your meal with the person. Eating with company can enhance mealtime abilities owing to social interaction and taking cues to eat from others. In addition you can help keep their focus on the meal and provide appropriate assistance if required to help maintain food intake. It can also help carers become more aware of individuals' likes, dislikes and preferences.

-   Eating together (family style) on small round tables, increasing social interaction through welcoming individuals to the dining room or using an informal activity before eating (for example flower arranging) may prompt better attention and meal behaviour.

*   CARE HOME SPECIFIC: Increase socialisation:

    -   Consider who the person is sitting with or who is sat around them. Try to identify whether they do not like sitting near or next to other people and change seating arrangements to avoid any problems. Sit the person with a friend or someone they have an affinity with to enhance social interaction, which may improve the meal behaviour by increasing stimulation (rather than seating based on assistance needs).

*   REFERRAL: Check and rule out any underlying physical problems; for example complete a pain assessment or speak to the person's doctor to investigate any medication-related side effects.

12

Summary and Conclusions

Overview

Mealtimes for people with dementia are critical not only for the need to consume adequate food and fluid but also to preserve dignity and personhood through familiar rituals and social interaction (Aselage and Amella, 2010). The mealtime care of the person with mid- to later-stage dementia is complex (Durnbaugh *et al.*, 1996) and is one of the most challenging and time-consuming roles in a carer's day (Aselage and Amella, 2010).

There needs to be a priority on the earlier detection of reduced mealtime abilities. This will enable carers to implement multicomponent interventions to prevent conditions such as malnutrition impacting on someone's overall wellbeing (Steele *et al.*, 1997). There is a demand for people with dementia to enjoy a better mealtime experience which involves supporting their retained eating and social abilities to ensure they maintain independence and dignity at mealtimes.

Educational resources for family carers and care staff are needed to promote best practice in the mealtime care of people with dementia (Aselage and Amella, 2010). When carers are provided with the resources to identify reduced and retained mealtime abilities, then person-centred care plans can be produced to strengthen and support the person at mealtimes.

Adequate nutrition and hydration

Decreased food intake and the risk of malnutrition are common in people with dementia, although addressing this problem has been neglected in research and in practice (Prince *et al.*, 2014). As dementia advances and symptoms become more severe, increased weight loss

238

is observed and this pattern is repeated around the world (Albanese *et al.*, 2013).

The causes of weight loss are complex and depend on a number of factors but in the later stages of dementia the reduction in eating and drinking abilities and changes in meal behaviours have an important role to play. Indeed weight loss and reduced mealtime abilities are predictors of mortality in later-stage dementia, as they are in older people without dementia, and are particularly noticeable among the frail (Prince *et al.*, 2014). There is a link between weight loss and a low body mass index (BMI), and severely reduced mealtime abilities and behaviours (Smith and Greenwood, 2008).

As such it is recommended that for those at risk of decreased food intake and weight loss to be assessed for a range of mealtime abilities and have nutrition-based interventions implemented (Prince *et al.*, 2014).

Mealtime abilities

Reduced eating and drinking abilities and meal behaviours, referred to collectively in this book as mealtime abilities, are common as dementia progresses (Lin *et al.*, 2010). Reduced mealtime abilities have a major impact on decreased food and fluid intake, and physical and mental health, and often coincide with increased mealtime assistance usually provided in the form of feeding (Chang and Roberts, 2008). Trying to manage these changes in these abilities causes anxiety and strain for both family carers and care staff (Prince *et al.*, 2014). Mealtime ability varies from person to person; therefore assessment is required by carers to detect what strengths in mealtime abilities are retained and to provide more effective and suitable support through person-centred interventions for those abilities that are reduced (Lee and Song, 2015).

Person-centred Mealtime Dementia Care

The complexities of providing effective person-centred mealtime care for people living with dementia are slowly becoming better understood. It is very encouraging to see recent research highlighting the importance of multicomponent interventions to address the range of complexities discussed in this book, including: social interactions at mealtime; self-feeding ability; the dining environment; the attitudes, knowledge and skills of staff; adequate time to eat and availability of staff to provide assistance; sensory properties of the food; hospitality and mealtime logistics; choice and variety in the dining experience; and nutrient density of food (Keller *et al.*, 2015).

Assessment

A lack of both proper assessment and the knowledge to implement effective interventions can lead to a progressive loss of mealtime abilities for people living with dementia (Aselage and Amella, 2010). Assessment of mealtime abilities is crucial if carers are to understand the nutritional needs of those with later-stage dementia (Durnbaugh *et al.*, 1996).

The assessment of the person with dementia must encompass the mealtime. While currently people with dementia may be regularly weighed for weight loss and screened for malnutrition, and staff may complete food record charts, the assessment of mealtime abilities is non-existent. Screening for malnutrition in general is important but this screening does not provide information as to why someone has become malnourished or what interventions to implement. Indeed without timely and effective intervention once someone with dementia is malnourished, interventions become less effective and it becomes difficult to reverse malnutrition (Shatenstein *et al.*, 2008).

A complete lack of accessible tools to help identify abilities a person with dementia has at a mealtime does not help. This book has provided one option in the Dementia Mealtime Assessment Tool, which is also freely available online (DMAT, 2017).

It is important to accurately assess mealtime abilities in all people with dementia who require care, otherwise those who need support may get missed. Those with many retained mealtime abilities tend to eat independently and those with severely reduced mealtime abilities may receive full feeding assistance, while those with only a few or several reduced mealtime abilities and moderate dependency can be ignored (Lin *et al.*, 2010). Someone may be capable of feeding themselves but without the right support can struggle using cutlery or identifying food on the plate. In a busy mealtime environment they may go unnoticed as carers are preoccupied with feeding someone else. Or indeed these needs may go unnoticed due to lack of awareness and assessment, and gradually they lose weight and their eating abilities deteriorate further until they lose independence and are fed.

Often increased feeding assistance is provided without any assessment of the reasons for providing it (Berkhout *et al.*, 1998). The missed assessment of mealtime abilities prior to the person requiring full feeding assistance may not been recognised and neither might the implementation of interventions at this stage (Steele *et al.*, 1997). Therefore how do we know if other interventions could have been put in place to help the person continue to eat by themselves for longer?

If carers view people with dementia as dependent then they will provide care based on that belief. This means using costly and labour-intensive interventions such as feeding rather than supporting and empowering the person with dementia. Carers should not assume that mealtime abilities will continue to be lost: effort should be focused on retaining abilities rather than 'overcoming' disabilities. Importantly reduced mealtime abilities can be reacquired through person-centred interventions (Coyne and Hoskins, 1997).

Multicomponent interventions

Until further research helps us better understand what the most effective interventions are at improving a range of health outcomes, carers must ensure they are trying all they can to improve mealtime dementia care. It is imperative to harness the accumulative effects of several interventions. This book highlights many interventions that can be put in place to support mealtime care and provides a systematic approach to implementing multiple interventions. Hopefully having these multiple interventions readily available will help change attitudes and beliefs towards mealtime care of people with dementia. We must change the attitude of carers who feel mealtime care cannot be improved for people with later-stage dementia. When someone is not eating the old attitude presented of 'There's not much we can do' should be replaced with a 'Look how much we can try' attitude.

It is recommended that more importance should be placed on interventions that optimise social activity at mealtimes and that an increase in socialisation should be a core aspect of person-centred care (Prince *et al.*, 2014). A more familiar way of eating such as 'family-style' eating where food is served at the table rather than pre-plated can increase interactions between people with dementia and their carers. This type of approach has led to increased food intake and body weight along with quality of life. Importantly this type of intervention seems to work best in those with a low BMI who are in the later stages of dementia and therefore the most vulnerable. Carers eating their meals with the person with dementia can have similar positive effects and both interventions help foster person-centred care (Prince *et al.*, 2014).

Finally it is imperative that this assessment and multiple interventions are incorporated into a care plan which all carers are aware of and which can be monitored.

Care plans

Categorising meal behaviours and eating abilities is an essential first step to enable ways to plan and implement interventions to support the range of mealtime abilities. Neither the assessment nor interventions need be difficult or costly to implement.

A very useful and practical study involving people with advanced dementia looked at whether the duties carried out by carers in care homes were what was being documented in the care plans (Ullrich and McCutcheon, 2008). Unsurprisingly the care plans did not accurately reflect or represent the specific interventions carried out by carers. Carers provided many interventions but were not always recording them on the care plan; therefore different carers used different interventions, impacting on standards of care. Practically this meant only some carers were aware of the best practices to use to help support an individual's mealtime abilities and meal behaviours. Communication among care staff is often reliant on handovers and what is documented in the care plan. Changes in carers or having several different carers, or even new carers with a lack of training and experience in dementia care or knowledge of the people they are caring for, create more difficulties (Ullrich and McCutcheon, 2008). These carers may be unaware how to support the person without some prompting or guidance; if what to do when, for example, they refuse to eat or have other reduced mealtime abilities is not documented in the care plan, then the person, will not be supported appropriately.

Accuracy in recording the many simple and complex caring techniques used to provide better mealtime care is required. This is no simple task but by using a structured process such as outlined in this book carers can record and monitor the complex mealtime care they provide in a practical care plan.

Training and resources

Carers currently have no specific training on identifying mealtime abilities. There is a need to provide staff with information on assessing changing mealtime needs and implementing interventions for supporting mealtime abilities (Lin *et al.*, 2010). In particular unpaid or informal carers lack the information, resources and support needed to help their family members eat adequately (Shatenstein *et al.*, 2008).

Training and education regarding common mealtime abilities in mid- to later-stage dementia and how carers can enhance the environment, meal presentation and their interaction with the people they care for may also increase the focus of mealtime care in this at-risk and vulnerable group (Durnbaugh *et al.*, 1996). Furthermore the assessment of mealtime abilities can help guide and develop appropriate training programmes to maintain or improve their remaining mealtime abilities and can be combined with changes to the physical and social environment (Lee and Song, 2015).

Research has shown that training staff to use many of the interventions suggested in this book can improve food intake at mealtimes (Batchelor-Murphy *et al.*, 2015a). Ideally a combination of training and practical experience using the mealtime interventions described may help to achieve improved mealtime abilities and nutritional outcomes.

To conclude

At the present time there is no cure for dementia. More research needs to focus on creating evidence-based best practices for very real and everyday caring needs such as mealtimes which promote person-centred care and quality of life.

The mealtime care for people living with dementia, especially as the disease progresses, must become more than just focusing on the consumption of food for calories and to maintain weight. They must encompass the experience of social activity and link appropriately with culture and background. Meals occur at least three times a day and can last more than one hour, and therefore play a crucial role in everyday life.

Dementia affects the ability to eat and drink and increases behavioural symptoms experienced at mealtimes. Reduced mealtime abilities lead to a loss of independence while eating, decreased food and fluid intake (with associated malnutrition) and negative impact on dignity – all resulting in reduced quality of life and wellbeing.

Retaining and enhancing mealtime abilities is therefore an essential part of nutrition care for people living with dementia. Carers are required to provide complex care with the emphasis at mealtimes on supporting mealtime abilities. Using a person-centred approach can not only improve on this but also promote a sense of self and self-worth in the people being cared for.

Resources to help carers achieve this are lacking and it is hoped that this book can provide carers with one practical resource to expand their caring knowledge and skills.

References

Abbott, R.A., Whear, R., Thompson-Coon, J., Ukoumunne, O.C. *et al.* (2013) 'Effectiveness of mealtime interventions on nutritional outcomes for the elderly living in residential care: A systematic review and meta-analysis', *Ageing Research Reviews*, 12(4), pp. 967–981. doi: 10.1016/j.arr.2013.06.002.

Abdelhamid, A., Bunn, D.K., Dickinson, A., Killett, A. *et al.* (2016) 'Effectiveness of interventions to improve, maintain or facilitate oral food and/or drink intake in people with dementia: Systematic review', *BMC Geriatrics*, 14(Suppl 2), p. P1. doi: 10.1186/1472-6963-14-S2-P1.

ADA (American Dietetic Association) (2005) 'Position of the American Dietetic Association: Liberalization of the diet prescription improves quality of life for older adults in long-term care', *Journal of the American Dietetic Association*, 105(12), pp. 1955–1965. doi: 10.1016/j.jada.2005.10.004.

Adam, H. and Preston, A.J. (2006) 'The oral health of individuals with dementia in nursing homes', *Gerodontology*, 23(2), pp. 99–105. doi: 10.1111/j.1741-2358.2006.00118.x.

Alagiakrishnan, K., Bhanji, R.A. and Kurian, M. (2013) 'Evaluation and management of oropharyngeal dysphagia in different types of dementia: A systematic review', *Archives of Gerontology and Geriatrics*, 56(1), pp. 1–9. doi: 10.1016/j.archger.2012.04.011.

Albanese, E., Taylor, C., Siervo, M., Stewart, R., Prince, M.J. and Acosta, D. (2013) 'Dementia severity and weight loss: A comparison across eight cohorts. The 10/66 study', *Alzheimer's & Dementia: The Journal of the Alzheimer's Association*, 9(6), pp. 649–656. doi: 10.1016/j.jalz.2012.11.014.

Algase, D.L., Beck, C., Kolanowski, A., Whall, A. *et al.* (1996) 'Need-driven dementia-compromised behavior: An alternative view of disruptive behavior', *American Journal of Alzheimer's Disease*, 11(6), pp. 10–19. Available at: http://journals.sagepub.com/doi/abs/10.1177/153331759601100603 (Accessed: 3 July 2018).

Alibhai, S.M.H., Greenwood, C. and Payette, H. (2005) 'An approach to the management of unintentional weight loss in elderly people', *Canadian Medical Association Journal*, 172(6), pp. 773–780. doi: 10.1503/cmaj.1031527.

Allen, V.J., Methven, L. and Gosney, M.A. (2013) 'Use of nutritional complete supplements in older adults with dementia: Systematic review and meta-analysis of clinical outcomes', *Clinical Nutrition*, 32(6), pp. 950–957. doi: 10.1016/j.clnu.2013.03.015.

Alzheimer's Association (2017) 'Stages of Alzheimer's'. Available at: www.alz.org/alzheimers_disease_stages_of_alzheimers.asp (Accessed: 3 July 2018).

Alzheimer's Australia (2015) 'Dementia Language Guidelines'. Available at: www. fightdementia.org.au/files/NATIONAL/documents/language-guidelines-full.pdf (Accessed: 3 July 2018).

Alzheimer's Australia (2017) 'Progression of dementia'. Available at: www.fightdementia. org.au/about-dementia/what-is-dementia/progression-of-dementia (Accessed: 3 July 2018).

Alzheimer's Society (2009) 'Person-centred care'. Available at: www.alzheimers.org.uk/ info/20009/treatments/159/person-centred_care (Accessed: 3 July 2018).

Alzheimer's Society (2016) 'Dental care'. Available at: www.alzheimers.org.uk/site/ scripts/documents_info.php?documentID=138 (Accessed: 3 July 2018).

Alzheimer's Society (2017) 'The later stages of dementia'. Available at: www.alzheimers. org.uk/info/20073/how_dementia_progresses/103/the_later_stages_of_ dementia (Accessed: 3 July 2018).

Amella, E.J. (1999) 'Factors influencing the proportion of food consumed by nursing home residents with dementia', *Journal of the American Geriatrics Society*, 47(7), pp. 879–885. Available at: www.ncbi.nlm.nih.gov/pubmed/10404936 (Accessed: 3 July 2018).

Armstrong, R.A. (2009) 'Alzheimer's disease and the eye', *Journal of Optometry*, 2(3), pp. 103–111. doi: 10.3921/joptom.2009.103.

Arrighi, H.M., Neumann, P.J., Lieberburg, I.M. and Townsend, R.J. (2010) 'Lethality of Alzheimer Disease and its impact on nursing home placement', *Alzheimer Disease & Associated Disorders*, 24(1), pp. 90–95. doi: 10.1097/WAD.0b013e31819fe7d1.

Aselage, M.B. (2010) 'Measuring mealtime difficulties: Eating, feeding and meal behaviours in older adults with dementia', *Journal of Clinical Nursing*, 19(5–6), pp. 621–631. doi: 10.1111/j.1365-2702.2009.03129.x.

Aselage, M.B. and Amella, E.J. (2010) 'An evolutionary analysis of mealtime difficulties in older adults with dementia', *Journal of Clinical Nursing*, 19(1–2), pp. 33–41. doi: 10.1111/j.1365-2702.2009.02969.x.

Aselage, M. and Amella, E. (2012) 'Response to Watson R (2011) Commentary on Aselage MB (2010) Measuring mealtime difficulties: Eating, feeding, and meal behaviours in older adults with dementia. Journal of Clinical Nursing 19, 621–631. Journal of Clinical Nursing 20, 297–298', *Journal of Clinical Nursing*, 21(9–10), pp. 1494–1495. doi: 10.1111/j.1365-2702.2012.04072.x.

Aselage, M.B., Amella, E.J. and Watson, R. (2011) 'State of the science: Alleviating mealtime difficulties in nursing home residents with dementia', *Nursing Outlook*, 59(4), pp. 210–214. doi: 10.1016/j.outlook.2011.05.009.

Bannerman, E. and McDermott, K. (2011) 'Dietary and fluid intakes of older adults in care homes requiring a texture-modified diet: The role of snacks', *Journal of the American Medical Directors Association*, 12(3), pp. 234–239. doi: 10.1016/j. jamda.2010.06.001.

Batchelor-Murphy, M.K., Amella, E.J., Zapka, J., Mueller, M. *et al.* (2015a) 'Feasibility of a web-based dementia feeding skills training program for nursing home staff', *Geriatric Nursing*, 36(3), pp. 212–218. doi: 10.1016/j.gerinurse.2015.02.003.

Batchelor-Murphy, M.K., Amella, E.J., Anderson, R.A., McConnell, E. *et al.* (2015b) 'Fidelity to treatment: Implementing an experimental comparison of dementia hand feeding techniques', *The Gerontologist*, 55(2), p. 85.

Batchelor-Murphy, M.K., Amella, E., Anderson, R., McConnell, E.S. *et al.* (2016) 'Supportive hand feeding in dementia: Establishing evidence for three hand feeding techniques', in *27th International Nursing Research Congress*. Available at: www. nursinglibrary.org/vhl/handle/10755/616136 (Accessed: 3 July 2018).

Batchelor-Murphy, M.K., McConnell, E.S., Amella, E.J., Anderson, R.A. *et al.* (2017) 'Experimental comparison of efficacy for three handfeeding techniques in dementia', *Journal of the American Geriatrics Society*, 65(4), pp. e89–e94. doi: 10.1111/jgs.14728.

BDA (British Dental Association) (2013) 'Dental problems and their management in patients with dementia'. Available at: www.bda.org/dentists/education/sgh/ Documents/Dental problems and their management in patients with dementia.pdf (Accessed: 3 July 2018).

Berkhout, A.M.M., Cools, H.J.M. and Van Houwelingen, H.C. (1998) 'The relationship between difficulties in feeding oneself and loss of weight in nursing-home patients with dementia', *Age and Ageing*, 27(5), pp. 637–641. doi: 10.1093/ageing/27.5.637.

Britton, B. (2012) 'Hard to swallow'. Available at: http://d4dementia.blogspot.com. es/2012/09/hard-to-swallow.html (Accessed: 3 July 2018).

Britton, B. (2015) 'The stages of dementia'. Available at: http://d4dementia.blogspot. co.uk/2015/11/the-stages-of-dementia.html (Accessed: 3 July 2018).

Brooke, J. and Ojo, O. (2015) 'Oral and enteral nutrition in dementia: An overview', *British Journal of Nursing*, 24(12), pp. 624–628.

Brush, J.A. (2001) 'Improving dining for people with dementia', *Center for Architecture and Urban Planning Research Books: Book 17*. Available at: https://dc.uwm.edu/caupr_ mono/17 (Accessed 3 July 2018).

Brush, J. and Calkins, M. (2008) 'Environmental interventions and dementia: Enhancing mealtimes in group dining rooms', *The ASHA Leader*. Available at: http://leader.pubs. asha.org/article.aspx?articleid=2289752 (Accessed: 3 July 2018).

Brush, J., Meehan, R. and Calkins, M. (2002) 'Using the environment to improve intake for people with dementia', *Alzheimer's Care Quarterly*, 3(4), pp. 330–338. Available at: http://journals.lww.com/actjournalonline/Abstract/2002/03040/Using_the_ Environment_To_Improve_Intake_for_People.7.aspx (Accessed: 4 July 2018).

Brush, J.A., Fleder, H.A. and Calkins, M.P. (2012) 'Using the Environment to Support Communication and Foster Independence in People with Dementia'. Available at: www.ideasconsultinginc.com/pdfs/ideas_publication_may2012.pdf (Accessed: 3 July 2018).

Calkins, M.P. (2006) 'Dining room design', Dementia Design Info, p. 11. Available at: www4.uwm.edu/dementiadesigninfo/ (Accessed: 4 July 2018).

Calkins, M.P. (2010) 'Using color as a therapeutic tool', Ideas Institute. Available at: www. ideasinstitute.org/article_021103_b.asp (Accessed: 4 July 2018).

Chan, C.P.H. and Kwan, Y.K. (2014) 'Feeding-swallowing issues in older adults with dementia', *Asian Journal of Gerontology and Geriatrics*, 9(2), pp. 80–84.

Chang, C.-C. (2012) 'Prevalence and factors associated with feeding difficulty in institutionalized elderly with dementia in Taiwan', *Journal of Nutrition, Health & Aging*, 16(3), pp. 258–261. Available at: www.ncbi.nlm.nih.gov/pubmed/22456783 (Accessed: 4 July 2018).

Chang, C.-C. and Roberts, B.L. (2008) 'Feeding difficulty in older adults with dementia', *Journal of Clinical Nursing*, 17(17), pp. 2266–2274. doi: 10.1111/j.1365-2702.2007.02275.x.

Charras, K. and Frémontier, M. (2010) 'Sharing meals with institutionalized people with dementia: A natural experiment', *Journal of Gerontological Social Work*, 53(5), pp. 436–448. doi: 10.1080/01634372.2010.489936.

Chaudhury, H., Hung, L. and Badger, M. (2013) 'The role of physical environment in supporting person-centered dining in long-term care: A review of the literature', *American Journal of Alzheimer's Disease and Other Dementias*, 28(5), pp. 491–500. doi: 10.1177/1533317513488923.

Cichero, J.A. (2013) 'Thickening agents used for dysphagia management: Effect on bioavailability of water, medication and feelings of satiety', *Nutrition Journal*, 12(1), p. 54. doi: 10.1186/1475-2891-12-54.

Cichero, J.A.Y., Steele, C., Duivestein, J., Clavé, P. *et al.* (2013) 'The need for international terminology and definitions for texture-modified foods and thickened liquids used in dysphagia management: Foundations of a global initiative', *Current Physical Medicine and Rehabilitation Reports*, 1(4), pp. 280–291. doi: 10.1007/s40141-013-0024-z.

Cleary, S., Hopper, T. and Van Soest, D. (2012) 'Reminiscence therapy, mealtimes and improving intake in residents with dementia', *Canadian Nursing Home*, 23(2), p. 8. Available at: http://connection.ebscohost.com/c/articles/78386644/reminiscence-therapy-mealtimes-improving-intake-residents-dementia (Accessed: 4 July 2018).

Coduras, A., Rabasa, I., Frank, A., Bermejo-Pareja, F. *et al.* (2010) 'Prospective one-year cost-of-illness study in a cohort of patients with dementia of Alzheimer's disease type in Spain: The ECO study', *Journal of Alzheimer's Disease*, 19(2), pp. 601–615. doi: 10.3233/JAD-2010-1258.

Cohen-Mansfield, J. (2000) 'Theoretical frameworks for behavioral problems in dementia', *Alzheimer's Care Quarterly*, 1, pp. 8–21.

Coyne, M.L. and Hoskins, L. (1997) 'Improving eating behaviors in dementia using behavioral strategies', *Clinical Nursing Research*, 6(3), pp. 275–290. doi: 10.1177/105477389700600307.

Crawley, H. and Hocking, E. (2011) *Eating Well: Supporting Older People and Older People with Dementia*. Abbots Langley: The Caroline Walker Trust.

DEEP (Dementia Engagement and Empowerment Project) (2014) 'Dementia words matter: Guidelines on language about dementia'. Available at: http://dementiavoices.org.uk/wp-content/uploads/2015/03/DEEP-Guide-Language.pdf (Accessed: 4 July 2018).

DEEP (2015a) 'Dementia Care Environment Audit Tools & Services'. Available at: www.enablingenvironments.com.au/audit-tools--services.html (Accessed: 4 July 2018).

DEEP (2015b) 'Dining Area, Dementia Enabling Environments'. Available at: www.enablingenvironments.com.au/dining-areas.html (Accessed: 4 July 2018).

DEEP (2015c) 'Lighting audit tool' *(DEEP)*. Available at: www.enablingenvironments.com.au/uploads/5/0/4/5/50459523/lighting-audit-tool.pdf (Accessed: 4 July 2018).

Dementia UK (2017) 'Life Story Work'. Available at: www.dementiauk.org/for-healthcare-professionals/free-resources/life-story-work/ (Accessed: 4 July 2018).

Department of Health (2015) *Dementia-friendly Health and Social Care Environments*. Available at: https://assets.publishing.service.gov.uk/government/uploads/system/uploads/attachment_data/file/416780/HBN_08-02.pdf (Accessed: 4 July 2018).

Desai, J., Winter, A., Young, K.W.H. and Greenwood, C.E. (2007) 'Changes in type of foodservice and dining room environment preferentially benefit institutionalized seniors with low body mass indexes', *Journal of the American Dietetic Association*, 107(5), pp. 808–814. doi: 10.1016/j.jada.2007.02.018.

Dewing, J. (2009) 'Caring for people with dementia: Noise and light', *Nursing Older People*, 21(5), pp. 34–38. doi: 10.7748/nop2009.06.21.5.34.c7102.

DHSC (Department of Health and Social Care) and AHPPU (Allied Health Professions Policy Unit) (2016) *Making a Difference in Dementia: Nursing Vision and Strategy Refreshed Edition*. Available at: www.gov.uk/government/publications/dementia-nursing-vision-and-strategy (Accessed: 4 July 2018).

DMAT (2017) 'Dementia Mealtime Assessment Tool'. Available at: www.thedmat.com/ (Accessed: 4 July 2018).

DSDC (Dementia Services Development Centre) (2012a) 'The importance of lighting'. Available at: http://dementia.stir.ac.uk/design/virtual-environments/importance-design/importance-lighting (Accessed: 4 July 2018).

DSDC (2012b) 'Virtual Care Home'. Available at: http://dementia.stir.ac.uk/design/virtual-environments/virtual-care-home (Accessed: 4 July 2018).

Dunne, T.E., Neargarder, S.A., Cipolloni, P.B. and Cronin-Golomb, A. (2004) 'Visual contrast enhances food and liquid intake in advanced Alzheimer's disease.' *Clinical Nutrition*, 23(4), pp. 533–538.

Durnbaugh, T., Haley, B. and Roberts, S. (1996) 'Assessing problem feeding behaviors in mid-stage Alzheimer's disease', *Geriatric Nursing*, 17(2), pp. 63–67. Available at: https://www.gnjournal.com/article/S0197-4572(96)80170-4/pdf (Accessed: 27 July 2018).

Dutton, B. (2017) 'How to manage dysphagia', *Australian Journal of Dementia Care*, 6(4), pp. 21–25.

Dyer, S. and Greenwood, C. (2001) 'Consistency of breakfast consumption in institutionalised seniors with cognitive impairment: Its value and use in feeding programs', *Journal of American Geriatric Society*, 49(4), pp. 494–496.

Eberhardie, C. (2004) 'Assessment and management of eating skills in the older adult', *Nursing Times*. Available at: www.nursingtimes.net/roles/older-people-nurses/assessment-and-management-of-eating-skills-in-the-older-adult/199540.article (Accessed: 4 July 2018).

Ekberg, O., Hamdy, S., Woisard, V., Wuttge-Hannig, A. and Ortega, P. (2002) 'Social and psychological burden of dysphagia: Its impact on diagnosis and treatment', *Dysphagia*, 17(2), pp. 139–146. doi: 10.1007/s00455-001-0113-5.

Engstrom, G. and Marmstal Hammar, L. (2012) 'Humming as a potential tool for facilitating feeding situations between persons with dementia and their caregiver: A single case study', *Music and Medicine*, 4, pp. 231–236. doi: 10.1177/1943862112456042.

EPUT (Essex Partnership University NHS Foundation Trust) (2017) *Food First*. Available at: https://eput.nhs.uk/our-services/bedfordshire-and-luton/bedfordshire-community-health-services/adults/nutrition-dietetics/food-first (Accessed: 4 July 2018).

Farrer, O., Olsen, C., Mousley, K. and Teo, E. (2015) 'Does presentation of smooth pureed meals improve patients' consumption in an acute care setting? A pilot study', *Nutrition & Dietetics*. doi: 10.1111/1747-0080.12198.

Gilmore-Bykovskyi, A.L. (2015) 'Caregiver person-centeredness and behavioral symptoms during mealtime interactions: Development and feasibility of a coding scheme', *Geriatric Nursing*, 36(2), pp. S10–S15. doi: 10.1016/j.gerinurse.2015.02.018.

Griffin, A., Hollingworth, L., Tyberek, M., Vourgaslis, J., Czapnik, D. and Mcneill-brown, D. (2009) *Dining with Dementia*. Melbourne: La Trobe University. Available at: www.speech-therapy.com.au/assets/uploads/2016/02/Dining-with-Dementia-relating-to-dysphagia.pdf (Accessed: 4 July 2018).

Halton Region Health Department (2012) 'Oral Care for Individuals with Dementia'. Available at: www.halton.ca/common/pages/UserFile.aspx?fileId=100067 (Accessed: 4 July 2018).

Hammar, L.M., Swall, A. and Meranius, M.S. (2016) 'Ethical aspects of caregivers' experience with persons with dementia at mealtimes', *Nursing Ethics*, 23(6), pp. 624–635. doi: 10.1177/0969733015580812.

Hammond Care (2014) 'Cracking Recipes'. Available at: www.hammond.com.au/services/food-culture/dont-give-me-eggs-that-bounce (Accessed: 4 July 2018).

Hanson, L.C., Ersek, M., Gilliam, R. and Carey, T.S. (2011) 'Oral feeding options for people with dementia: A systematic review', *Journal of the American Geriatrics Society*, 59(3), pp. 463–472. doi: 10.1111/j.1532-5415.2011.03320.x.

Hanson, L.C., Ersek, M., Lin, F.C. and Carey, T.S. (2013) 'Outcomes of feeding problems in advanced dementia in a nursing home population', *Journal of the American Geriatrics Society*, 61(10), pp. 1692–1697. doi: 10.1111/jgs.12448.

Hardy, C.J.D., Marshall, C.R., Golden, H.L., Clark, C.N. *et al.* (2016) 'Hearing and dementia', *Journal of Neurology*, 263(11), pp. 2339–2354. doi: 10.1007/s00415-016-8208-y.

Herke, M., Burckhardt, M., Wustmann, T., Watzke, S., Fink, A. and Langer, G. (2015) 'Environmental and behavioural modifications for improving food and fluid intake in people with dementia', *Cochrane Database of Systematic Reviews*. doi: 10.1002/14651858.CD011542.

Hines, S., McCrow, J., Abbey, J. and Gledhill, S. (2010) 'Thickened fluids for people with dementia in residential aged care facilities', *International Journal of Evidence-Based Healthcare*, 8(4), pp. 252–255. doi: 10.1111/j.1744-1609.2010.00188.x.

Hsiao, H.-C., Chao, H.-C. and Wang, J.-J. (2013) 'Features of problematic eating behaviors among community-dwelling older adults with dementia: Family caregivers' experience', *Geriatric Nursing*, 34(5), pp. 361–365. doi: 10.1016/j.gerinurse.2013.06.010.

Hung, L., Chaudhury, H. and Rust, T. (2016) 'The effect of dining room physical environmental renovations on person-centered care practice and residents' dining experiences in long-term care facilities', *Journal of Applied Gerontology*, 35(12), pp. 1279–1301. doi: 10.1177/0733464815574094.

IDDSI (International Dysphagia Diet Standardization Initiative) (2016)'What is the IDDSI Framework?' Available at: http://iddsi.org/framework/ (Accessed: 4 July 2018).

Ikeda, M., Brown, J., Holland, A.J., Fukuhara, R. and Hodges, J.R. (2002) 'Changes in appetite, food preference, and eating habits in frontotemporal dementia and Alzheimer's disease', *Journal of Neurology, Neurosurgery, and Psychiatry*, 73, pp. 371–376.

Jakob, A. and Collier, L. (2013) 'How to make a Sensory Room for people living with dementia: A Guide Book', p. 70. doi: 10.13140/2.1.1864.5283. Available at http://eprints.kingston.ac.uk/30132/1/Jakob-A-29602.pdf (Accessed: 4 July 2018).

Jansen, S., Ball, L., Desbrow, B., Morgan, K., Moyle, W. and Hughes, R. (2015) 'Nutrition and dementia care: Informing dietetic practice', *Nutrition & Dietetics*, 72(1), pp. 36–46. doi: 10.1111/1747-0080.12144.

Joliffe, J. and Chadwick, D. (2006) 'Guide to levels of risk of negative health consequences from dysphagia'. Available at: www.choiceforum.org/docs/dysphriska.doc (Accessed: 27 July 2018).

Kane, M. and Terry, G. (2015) 'Dementia 2015: Aiming higher to transform lives'. Available at: https://www.alzheimers.org.uk/sites/default/files/migrate/downloads/dementia_2015_aiming_higher_to_transform_lives.pdf (Accessed: 4 July 2018).

Keller, H.H. (2016) 'Improving food intake in persons living with dementia', *Annals of the New York Academy of Sciences*, 1367(1), pp. 3–11. doi: 10.1111/nyas.12997.

Keller, H.H., Gibbs-Ward, A., Randall-Simpson, J., Bocock, M.A. and Dimou, E. (2006) 'Meal rounds: An essential aspect of quality nutrition services in long-term care', *Journal of the American Medical Directors Association*, 7(1), pp. 40–45. doi: 10.1016/j.jamda.2005.06.009.

Keller, H., Beck, A.M. and Namasivayam, A. (2015) 'Improving food and fluid intake for older adults living in long-term care: A research agenda', *Journal of the American Medical Directors Association*, 16(2), pp. 93–100. doi: 10.1016/j.jamda.2014.10.017.

Kellett, R. (2012) *Communication and Mealtimes Toolkit: Helping people with dementia to eat, drink & communicate: A guide for carers.* Available at: http://www.nhsdg.scot.nhs.uk/Departments_and_Services/Speech_and_Language_Therapy/Adult_SLT/Documents/Communication___Mealtimes_Toolkit_for_Dementia_2013.pdf (Accessed 4 July 2018).

King's Fund (2014) 'Is your care home dementia friendly? EHE Environmental Assessment Tool.' Available at: www.kingsfund.org.uk/sites/files/kf/field/field_pdf/is-your-care-home-dementia-friendly-ehe-tool-kingsfund-mar13.pdf (Accessed: 4 July 2018).

Kovach, C.R., Noonan, P.E., Schlidt, A.M. and Wells, T. (2005) 'A model of consequences of need-driven, dementia-compromised behavior', *Journal of Nursing Scholarship*, 37(2), p. 134–140; discussion 140. Available at: http://www.ncbi.nlm.nih.gov/pubmed/15960057 (Accessed: 4 July 2018).

LeClerc, C.M., Wells, D.L., Sidani, S., Dawson, P. and Fay, J. (2004) 'A feeding abilities assessment for persons with dementia', *Alzheimer's Care Quarterly*, 5(2), pp. 123–133.

Lee, K.M. and Song, J.A. (2015) 'Factors influencing the degree of eating ability among people with dementia', *Journal of Clinical Nursing*, 24(11–12), pp. 1707–1717. doi: 10.1111/jocn.12777.

Leslie, W.S., Woodward, M., Lean, M.E.J., Theobald, H., Watson, L. and Hankey, C.R. (2013) 'Improving the dietary intake of under-nourished older people in residential care homes using an energy-enriching food approach: A cluster-randomised controlled study', *Journal of Human Nutrition and Dietetics*, 26(4), pp. 387–394. doi: 10.1111/jhn.12020.

Life Changes Trust (2015) 'Dementia and Sensory Challenges'. Available at: http://www.lifechangestrust.org.uk/sites/default/files/Leaflet.pdf (Accessed: 4 July 2018).

Lin, L.-C., Watson, R. and Wu, S.-C. (2010) 'What is associated with low food intake in older people with dementia?', *Journal of Clinical Nursing*, 19(1–2), pp. 53–59. doi: 10.1111/j.1365-2702.2009.02962.x.

Lindroos, E., Saarela, R.K.T., Soini, H., Muurinen, S., Suominen, M.H. and Pitkälä, K.H. (2014) 'Caregiver-reported swallowing difficulties, malnutrition, and mortality among older people in assisted living facilities', *Journal of Nutrition, Health & Aging*, 18(7), pp. 718–722. doi: 10.1007/s12603-014-0467-7.

Liu, M.F., Miao, N.F., Chen, I.H., Lin, Y.K. *et al.* (2015) 'Development and psychometric evaluation of the Chinese Feeding Difficulty Index (Ch-FDI) for people with dementia', *PLoS ONE*, 10(7), pp. 1–10. doi: 10.1371/journal.pone.0133716.

Liu, W., Cheon, J. and Thomas, S.A. (2014) 'Interventions on mealtime difficulties in older adults with dementia: A systematic review', *International Journal of Nursing Studies*, 51(1), pp. 14–27. doi: 10.1016/j.ijnurstu.2012.12.021.

Liu, W., Galik, E., Boltz, M., Nahm, E.-S. and Resnick, B. (2015) 'Optimizing eating performance for older adults with dementia living in long-term care: A systematic review', *Worldviews on Evidence-Based Nursing*, 12(4), pp. 228–235. doi: 10.1111/wvn.12100.

Maitre, I., Van Wymelbeke, V., Amand, M., Vigneau, E., Issanchou, S. and Sulmont-Rossé, C. (2014) 'Food pickiness in the elderly: Relationship with dependency and malnutrition', *Food Quality and Preference*, 32(Part B), pp. 145–151. doi: 10.1016/j.foodqual.2013.04.003.

Mamhidir, A.G., Karlsson, I., Norberg, A. and Mona, K. (2007) 'Weight increase in patients with dementia, and alteration in meal routines and meal environment after integrity-promoting care', *Journal of Clinical Nursing*, 16(5), pp. 987–996. doi: 10.1111/j.1365-2702.2006.01780.x.

Martin, L. (2017) 'Oral nutritional supplements: Are they an effective intervention in people living with dementia?', *Network Health Digest*, pp. 19–24. Available at: https://issuu.com/nhpublishingltd/docs/issue_129_digital?e=14357770/54948663 (Accessed: 4 July 2018).

Matthews, F.E., Stephan, B.C.M., Robinson, L., Jagger, C., Barnes, L.E. and Arthur, A. (2016) 'A two-decade dementia incidence comparison from the Cognitive Function and Ageing Studies I and II', *Nature Communications*. doi: 10.1038/ncomms11398.

Milte, R., Shulver, W., Killington, M., Bradley, C., Miller, M. and Crotty, M. (2017) 'Struggling to maintain individuality: Describing the experience of food in nursing homes for people with dementia', *Archives of Gerontology and Geriatrics*, 72(May), pp. 52–58. doi: 10.1016/j.archger.2017.05.002.

Morgan-Jones, P., McIntosh, D., Greedy, L. and Ellis, P. (2016) *It's All About the Food Not the Fork! 107 Easy to Eat Meals in a Mouthful*. Sydney: HammondCare Media. Available at: www.hammond.com.au/shop/information-for-carers/its-all-about-the-food-not-the-fork (Accessed: 4 July 2018).

Murphy, J.L., Holmes, J. and Brooks, C. (2017) 'Nutrition and dementia care: Developing an evidence-based model for nutritional care in nursing homes', *BMC Geriatrics*, 17(1), p. 55. doi: 10.1186/s12877-017-0443-2.

National Food Service Management Institute (2005a) 'Chapter 5: Feeding Techniques, Adult Day Care Resource Manual for the USDA Child and Adult Care Food Program'. Available at: https://www.education.nh.gov/program/nutrition/documents/adultdaycareresourcemanual.pdf (Accessed: 27 July 2018).

National Food Service Management Institute (2005b) 'The Aging Process and Feeding Techniques, Adult Day Care Resources for the USDA Child and Adult Care Food Program'. Available at: https://fns-prod.azureedge.net/sites/default/files/CACFPAdult%20DayCareHandbook.pdf (Accessed: 27 July 2018).

Newman, R., Vilardell, N., Clavé, P. and Speyer, R. (2016) 'Effect of bolus viscosity on the safety and efficacy of swallowing and the kinematics of the swallow response in patients with oropharyngeal dysphagia: White Paper by the European Society for Swallowing Disorders (ESSD)', *Dysphagia*, 31(5), pp. 232–249. doi: 10.1007/s00455-016-9729-3.

NHS Choices (2015) 'Dementia guide – Symptoms of dementia'. Department of Health. Available at: www.nhs.uk/Conditions/dementia-guide/Pages/symptoms-of-dementia.aspx (Accessed: 4 July 2018).

NICE (National Institute for Health and Care Excellence) (2016) 'Oral health for adults in care homes NICE guideline [NG48]'. Available at: www.nice.org.uk/guidance/ng48 (Accessed: 4 July 2018).

Nijs, K.A.N.D., de Graaf, C., Kok, F.J. and van Staveren, W.A. (2006) 'Effect of family-style mealtimes on quality of life, physical performance, and body weight of nursing-home residents: Cluster randomised controlled trial', *British Medical Journal*, 332(7551), pp. 1180–1184. doi: 10.1136/bmj.38825.401181.7C.

NPSA (National Patient Safety Agency) (2011) 'Dysphagia Diet Food Texture Descriptors'. Available at: http://www.hospitalcaterers.org/media/1160/dysphagia-descriptors.pdf (Accessed: 4 July 2018).

O'Neil, M.E., Freeman, M., Christensen, V., Telerant, R., Addleman, A. and Kansagara, D. (2011) 'Evidence-based synthesis program: A systematic evidence review of non-pharmacological interventions for behavioral symptoms of dementia', *Health Services Research & Development*, p. 69. Available at https://www.hsrd.research.va.gov/publications/esp/dementia-nonpharm.pdf (Accessed: 4 July 2018).

ONS (Office for National Statistics) (2017) 'Deaths registered in England and Wales' (Series DR). Available at: www.ons.gov.uk/peoplepopulationandcommunity/births deathsandmarriages/deaths/bulletins/deathsregisteredinenglandandwales seriesdr/2015 (Accessed: 4 July 2018).

Osborn, C.L. and Marshall, M.J. (1993) 'Self-feeding performance in nursing home residents', *Journal of Gerontological Nursing*, 19(3), pp. 7–9. doi: 10.3928/0098-9134-19930301-04.

Parrott, M.D., Young, K.W.H. and Greenwood, C.E. (2006) 'Energy-containing nutritional supplements can affect usual energy intake postsupplementation in institutionalized seniors with probable Alzheimer's disease', *Journal of the American Geriatrics Society*, 54(9), pp. 1382–1387. doi: 10.1111/j.1532-5415.2006.00844.x.

Pasman, H.R.W., The, B.A.M., Onwuteaka-Philipsen, B.D., Van Der Wal, G. and Ribbe, M.W. (2003) 'Feeding nursing home patients with severe dementia: A qualitative study', *Journal of Advanced Nursing*, 42(3), pp. 304–311. doi: 10.1046/j.1365-2648.2003.02620.x.

Patients Association (2015) 'Survey of medicines related care of residents with dysphagia in care homes'. Available at: www.patientlibrary.net/tempgen/84874.pdf (Accessed: 4 July 2018).

Pelletier, C.A. (2005) 'Feeding beliefs of certified nurse assistants in the nursing home: A factor influencing practice', *Journal of Gerontological Nursing*, 31(7), pp. 5–10. Available at: http://www.ncbi.nlm.nih.gov/pubmed/16047954 (Accessed: 4 July 2018).

Pouyet, V., Giboreau, A., Benattar, L. and Cuvelier, G. (2014) 'Attractiveness and consumption of finger foods in elderly Alzheimer's disease patients', *Food Quality and Preference*, 34, pp. 62–69. doi: 10.1016/j.foodqual.2013.12.011.

Premier Foods (2014) 'Dysphagia and Dementia: Healthcare Solutions'. Available at: http://premierfoodservice.co.uk/wp-content/uploads/2014/10/Premier_Healthcare_Brochure_11803.pdf (Accessed: 4 July 2018).

Prince, M., Emiliano, A., Maëlenn, G. and Matthew, P. (2014) 'Nutrition and dementia: A review of available research', *Alzheimer's Disease International*. doi: 10.1155/2012/926082. Available at https://www.alz.co.uk/sites/default/files/pdfs/nutrition-and-dementia.pdf (Accessed: 4 July 2018).

Public Health England (2016) 'Health matters: Midlife approaches to reduce dementia risk.' Available at: www.gov.uk/government/publications/health-matters-midlife-approaches-to-reduce-dementia-risk/health-matters-midlife-approaches-to-reduce-dementia-risk (Accessed: 4 July 2018).

Ragneskog, H., Kihlgren, M., Karlsson, I. and Norberg, A. (1996) 'Dinner music for demented patients: Analysis of video-recorded observations', *Clinical Nursing Research*, 5(3), pp. 262–277.

Reed, P., Zimmerman, S., Sloane, P., Williams, C. and Boustani, M. (2005) 'Characteristics associated with low food and fluid intake in long-term care residents with dementia', *The Gerontologist*, 45(Suppl 1), pp. 74–80.

Reimer, H.D. and Keller, H.H. (2009) 'Mealtimes in nursing homes: Striving for person-centered care', *Journal of Nutrition for the Elderly*, 28(4), pp. 327–347. doi: 10.1080/01639360903417066.

Rivière, S., Gillette-Guyonnet, S., Andrieu, S., Nourhashemi, F. *et al.* (2002) 'Cognitive function and caregiver burden: Predictive factors for eating behaviour disorders in Alzheimer's disease', *International Journal of Geriatric Psychiatry*, 17(10), pp. 950–955. doi: 10.1002/gps.724.

RNIB Scotland (2012) 'Dementia and sight loss: Looking after your eyes'. Available at: www.rnib.org.uk/eye-health/sight-loss-other-medical-conditions/dementia-and-sight-loss (Accessed: 4 July 2018).

Schiffman, S.S. (1983) 'Taste and smell in disease', *New England Journal of Medicine*, 308(22), pp. 1337–1343.

Schiffman, S.S. and Graham, B.G. (2000) 'Taste and smell perception affect appetite and immunity in the elderly', *European Journal of Clinical Nutrition*, 54(Suppl 3), pp. S54-63. Available at: http://www.ncbi.nlm.nih.gov/pubmed/11041076 (Accessed: 4 July 2018).

Schiffman, S.S. and Warwick, Z.S. (1993) 'Effect of flavor enhancement of foods for the elderly on nutritional status: Food intake, biochemical indexes, and anthropometric measures', *Physiology & Behavior*, 53(2), pp. 395–402. doi: 10.1016/0031-9384(93)90224-4.

SCIE (Social Care Institute for Excellence) (2015a) 'Activities for people with dementia based around food'. Available at: www.scie.org.uk/dementia/living-with-dementia/eating-well/activities-around-food.asp (Accessed: 4 July 2018).

SCIE (2015b) 'Noise levels: Dementia-friendly environments'. Available at: www.scie.org.uk/dementia/supporting-people-with-dementia/dementia-friendly-environments/noise.asp (Accessed: 4 July 2018).

Shanley, C. and O'Loughlin, G. (2000) 'Dysphagia among nursing home residents: An assessment and management protocol', *Journal of Gerontological Nursing*, 26(8), pp. 35–48. Available at: www.ncbi.nlm.nih.gov/pubmed/11276612 (Accessed: 4 July 2018).

Shatenstein, B., Kergoat, M.-J., Reid, I. and Chicoine, M.E. (2008) 'Dietary intervention in older adults with early-stage Alzheimer dementia: Early lessons learned', *Journal of Nutrition, Health & Aging*, 12(7), pp. 461–469. doi: 10.1007/BF02982707.

Simmons, S.F., Osterweil, D. and Schnelle, J.F. (2001) 'Improving food intake in nursing home residents with feeding assistance: A staffing analysis', *Journals of Gerontology: Series A*, 56(12), pp. M790-4. doi: 10.1093/GERONA/56.12.M790.

Simmons, S.F., Zhuo, X. and Keeler, E. (2010) 'Cost-effectiveness of nutrition interventions in nursing home residents: A pilot intervention', *Journal of Nutrition, Health & Aging*, 14(5), pp. 367–372. doi: 10.1016/j.pestbp.2011.02.012.Investigations.

Sing For Your Life (2014) 'Singing improves appetite'. Available at: www.singforyourlife.org.uk/news/2014-singing-improves-appetite (Accessed: 4 July 2018).

Slaughter, S.E., Eliasziw, M., Morgan, D. and Drummond, N. (2011) 'Incidence and predictors of eating disability among nursing home residents with middle-stage dementia', *Clinical Nutrition*, 30(2), pp. 172–177. doi: 10.1016/j.clnu.2010.09.001.

Smith, K.L. and Greenwood, C.E. (2008) 'Weight loss and nutritional considerations in Alzheimer Disease', *Journal of Nutrition for the Elderly*, 27(3–4), pp. 381–403. doi: 10.1080/01639360802265939.

Speyer, R., Baijens, L., Heijnen, M. and Zwijnenberg, I. (2010) 'Effects of therapy in oropharyngeal dysphagia by speech and language therapists: A systematic review', *Dysphagia*, 25(1), pp. 40–65. doi: 10.1007/s00455-009-9239-7.

Steele, C.M., Greenwood, C., Ens, I., Robertson, C. and Seidman-Carlson, R. (1997) 'Mealtime difficulties in a home for the aged: Not just dysphagia', *Dysphagia*, 12(1), pp. 43–51. doi: 10.1007/PL00009517.

Steele, C.M., Rivera, T., Bernick, L. and Mortensen, L. (2007) 'Insights regarding mealtime assistance for individuals in long-term care: Lessons from a time of crisis', *Topics in Geriatric Rehabilitation*, 23(4), pp. 319–329. doi: 10.1097/01. TGR.0000299160.67740.44.

Stockdell, R. and Amella, E.J. (2008) 'The Edinburgh Feeding Evaluation in Dementia Scale', *American Journal of Nursing*, 108(8), pp. 46–54.

Stone, L. (2014) 'Eating/feeding issues in dementia: Improving the dining experience', *End of Life Journal*, 4(1), pp. 1–7. Available at: www.stchristophers.org.uk/wp-content/uploads/2015/10/practice-development-1.EoLJ_.Vol4_.No1_.Dementia. pdf (Accessed: 4 July 2018).

Sung, H.-C. and Chang, A.M. (2005) 'Use of preferred music to decrease agitated behaviours in older people with dementia: A review of the literature', *Journal of Clinical Nursing*, 14(9), pp. 1133–1140. doi: 10.1111/j.1365-2702.2005.01218.x.

Sura, L., Madhavan, A., Carnaby, G. and Crary, M.A. (2012) 'Dysphagia in the elderly: Management and nutritional considerations', *Clinical Interventions in Aging*, 7, pp. 287–298. doi: 10.2147/CIA.S23404.

Swaffer, K. (2014) 'Dementia: Stigma, language, and dementia-friendly', *Dementia*, 13(6), pp. 709–716. doi: 10.1177/1471301214548143.

Talking Mats (2017) 'Dementia and Mealtimes'. Available at: www.talkingmats.com/ dementia-and-mealtimes/ (Accessed: 4 July 2018).

Taylor, S. (2016) 'Dysphagia: What every dietitian must know about thickeners', *Network Health Digest*, pp. 31–36. Available at: https://issuu.com/nhpublishingltd/docs/ issue_112d_web_file_1/31?e=14357770/33895135 (Accessed: 4 July 2018).

Timlin, G. and Rysenbry, N. (2010) *Design for Dementia: Improving Dining and Bedroom Environments in Care Homes*. London: Helen Hamlyn Centre, Royal College of Art.

Tristani, M. (2016) 'Dysphagia in persons with dementia: The dual diagnosis challenge', *Perspectives of the ASHA Special Interest Groups*, 1(Part 3), pp. 105–116.

Tsikritzi, R., Wang, J., Collins, V.J., Allen, V.J. *et al.* (2015) 'The effect of nutrient fortification of sauces on product stability, sensory properties, and subsequent liking by older adults', *Journal of Food Science*, 80(5), pp. S1100–S1110. doi: 10.1111/1750-3841.12850.

Tully, M.W., Matrakas, K.L., Muir, J. and Musallam, K. (1997) 'The Eating Behavior Scale: A simple method of assessing functional ability in patients with Alzheimer's disease', *Journal of Gerontological Nursing*, 23(7), pp. 9–15. Available at: http://www.ncbi.nlm. nih.gov/pubmed/9287601 (Accessed: 4 July 2018).

Ullrich, S. and McCutcheon, H. (2008) 'Nursing practice and oral fluid intake of older people with dementia', *Journal of Clinical Nursing*, 17(21), pp. 2910–2919. doi: 10.1111/j.1365-2702.2007.02274.x.

University of Bradford (2017) 'Dementia Care Mapping'. Available at: www.brad.ac.uk/ health/dementia/dementia-care-mapping/ (Accessed: 4 July 2018).

Van Ittersum, K. and Wansink, B. (2012) 'Plate size and color suggestibility: The Delboeuf illusion's bias on serving and eating behavior', *Journal of Consumer Research*, 39(2), pp. 215–228. doi: 10.1086/662615.

Vink, A.C., Birks, J.S., Bruinsma, M.S. and Scholten, R.J.S. (2004) 'Music therapy for people with dementia', *Cochrane Database of Systematic Reviews*, (3), p. CD003477. doi: 10.1002/14651858.CD003477.pub2.

Vitale, C., Monteloni, C., Burke, L., Frazier-Rios, D. and Volicer, L. (2009) 'Strategies for improving care for patients with advanced dementia and eating problems: Optimizing care through physician and speech pathologist collaboration', *Annals of Long-Term Care*, 17(5), pp. 32–39.

Vogelzang, J.L. (2003) 'Dignity and dietary interventions for dementia', *Home Healthcare Nurse*, 21(1), pp. 40–42. Available at: www.ncbi.nlm.nih.gov/pubmed/12544462 (Accessed: 4 July 2018).

Volkert, D., Chourdakis, M., Faxen-Irving, G., Frühwald, T. *et al.* (2015) 'ESPEN guidelines on nutrition in dementia', *Clinical Nutrition (Edinburgh, Scotland)*, 34(6), pp. 1052–1073. doi: 10.1016/j.clnu.2015.09.004.

Vucea, V., Keller, H.H. and Ducak, K. (2014) 'Interventions for improving mealtime experiences in long-term care', *Journal of Nutrition in Gerontology & Geriatrics*, 33(4), pp. 249–324. doi: 10.1080/21551197.2014.960339.

Walton, K., Williams, P., Tapsell, L., Hoyle, M. *et al.* (2013) 'Observations of mealtimes in hospital aged care rehabilitation wards', *Appetite*, 67, pp. 16–21. doi: 10.1016/j.appet.2013.03.006.

Watson, R. (1996) 'The Mokken scaling procedure (MSP) applied to the measurement of feeding difficulty in elderly people with dementia', *International Journal of Nursing Studies*, 33(4), pp. 385–393. doi: 10.1016/0020-7489(95)00058-5.

Watson, R. (2003) 'Response to feeding nursing home patients with severe dementia: A qualitative study', *Journal of Advanced Nursing*, 42(3), pp. 312–313. doi: 10.1111/j.1365-2648.2009.05201.x.

Watson, R. (2010) 'Commentary on Aselage MB (2010) Measuring mealtime difficulties: Eating, feeding and meal behaviour in older adults with dementia. Journal of clinical nursing 19, 621-631', *Journal of Clinical Nursing*, 19(19–20), pp. 2950–2951. doi: 10.1111/j.1365-2702.2010.03464.x.

Watson, R. and Green, S.M. (2006) 'Feeding and dementia: A systematic literature review', *Journal of Advanced Nursing*, 54(1), pp. 86–93. doi: 10.1111/j.1365-2648.2006.03793.x.

Weekes, C.E. (2008) 'The effect of protected mealtimes on meal interruptions, feeding assistance, energy and protein intake and plate waste', *Proceedings of the Nutrition Society*, 67(OCE/E119). doi: 10.1017/S0029665108007519.

Weijenberg, R.A.F., Lobbezoo, F., Knol, D.L., Tomassen, J. and Scherder, E.J.A. (2013) 'Increased masticatory activity and quality of life in elderly persons with dementia: A longitudinal matched cluster randomized single-blind multicenter intervention study', *BMC Neurology*, 13(1), p. 26. doi: 10.1186/1471-2377-13-26.

Whear, R., Abbott, R., Thompson-Coon, J., Bethel, A. *et al.* (2014) 'Effectiveness of mealtime interventions on behavior symptoms of people with dementia living in care homes: A systematic review', *Journal of the American Medical Directors Association*, 15(3), pp. 185–193. doi: 10.1016/j.jamda.2013.10.016.

WHO (World Health Organization) (2017) 'Dementia Key Facts'. Available at: www.who.int/news-room/fact-sheets/detail/dementia (Accessed: 4 July 2018).

Woodbridge, R., Sullivan, M., Harding, E., Crutch, S. *et al.* (2018) 'Use of the physical environment to support everyday activities for people with dementia: A systematic review', *Dementia*, 17(5), pp. 1–40. doi: 10.1177/1471301216648670.

Wright, L., Cotter, D., Hickson, M. and Frost, G. (2005) 'Comparison of energy and protein intakes of older people consuming a texture-modified diet with a normal hospital diet', *Journal of Human Nutrition and Dietetics*, 18(3), pp. 213–279. doi: 10.1111/j.1365-277X.2005.00605.x.

Wu, H.-S. and Lin, L.-C. (2015) 'Comparing cognition, mealtime performance, and nutritional status in people with dementia with or without ideational apraxia', *Biological Research for Nursing*, 17(2), pp. 199–206. doi: 10.1177/1099800414536773.

Young, K.W. H. and Greenwood, C.E. (2001) 'Shift in diurnal feeding patterns in nursing home residents with Alzheimer's disease', *Journals of Gerontology Series A: Biological Sciences and Medical Sciences*, 56(11), pp. M700–M706. doi: 10.1093/gerona/56.11.M700.

Young, K.W. H., Binns, M.A. and Greenwood, C.E. (2001) 'Meal delivery practices do not meet needs of Alzheimer patients with increased cognitive and behavioral difficulties in a long-term care facility', *Journal of Gerontology*, 56(10), pp. 656–661.

Young, K.W.H., Greenwood, C.E., Van Reekum, R. and Binns, M.A. (2004) 'Providing nutrition supplements to institutionalized seniors with probable Alzheimer's disease is least beneficial to those with low body weight status', *Journal of the American Geriatrics Society*, 52(8), pp. 1305–1312. doi: 10.1111/j.1532-5415.2004.52360.x.

Young, K.W.H., Greenwood, C., Van Reekum, R. and Binns, M. (2005) 'A randomized, crossover trial of high-carbohydrate foods in nursing home residents with Alzheimer's disease: Associations among intervention response, body mass index, behavioural and cognitive function', *Journal of Gerontology*, 60A(8), pp. 1039–1045.

Subject Index

Author Index